the
pregnancy
instruction
manual

[first trimester]

[second trimester]

[third trimester]

[congratulations!]

the
pregnancy
instruction manual

ESSENTIAL INFORMATION, TROUBLESHOOTING TIPS, AND ADVICE FOR PARENTS-TO-BE

by Sarah Jordan, with David Ufberg, M.D.

Illustrated by Paul Kepple and Scotty Reifsnyder

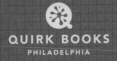

QUIRK BOOKS
PHILADELPHIA

Copyright © 2008 by Quirk Productions, Inc.

Illustrations copyright © 2008 by Headcase Design

All rights reserved. No part of this book may be reproduced in any form without written permission from the publisher.

Library of Congress Cataloging in Publication Number: 2008923025

ISBN: 978-1-59474-245-3

Printed in China

Typeset in Swiss

Design and illustrations by Paul Kepple and Scotty Reifsnyder @ Headcase Design
www.headcasedesign.com
Edited by Mindy Brown

Distributed in North America by Chronicle Books
680 Second Street
San Francisco, CA 94107

10 9 8 7 6 5 4 3 2 1

Quirk Books
215 Church Street
Philadelphia, PA 19106
www.quirkbooks.com

Contents

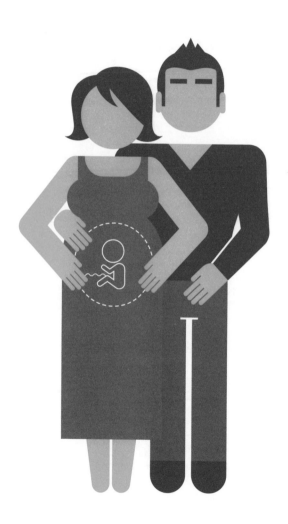

Welcome
to Your New
Pregnant Body!

Congratulations on your pregnancy!

The exhilaration of bringing a baby into the world is one of life's defining moments. It is a time of wonderment and joy, relief and pleasure to be able once again to sleep on your back and be heartburn free.

But there's no getting around it: Being pregnant can feel overwhelming. There is so much to learn and prepare for, and the myriad bizarre changes the body undergoes may make some women believe that something is surely amiss. How could all this peeing, palpitating, leakage, hemorrhoidal growth, sleepiness, crabbiness, and gassiness be normal? Well, it is. And you are about to become a veritable catalog of exaggerated bodily functions and fluids. It is all good preparation to desensitize you to the baby, who will display heroic disinhibition about his or her own bodily functions.

For women who want to do everything "right" for their baby, sweat every last detail, and leave no timely preparation undone, pregnancy can feel like the ultimate take-home exam where nothing less than an A+ will do. Believe us, by the time you're holding that baby in your arms, you may feel as knowledgeable as the resident who did your pelvic exam.

Fortunately, pregnancy runs on an automatic loop—building the baby from start to finish and then sending it out into the world when it's ready. You do not have to actually *do* anything to assemble the baby. You need not concern yourself with such questions as "How do I build an eye?" or "Am I creating a tip-top vestibular system?" or "Will my cervix know to contract the ten centimeters after the baby is delivered?" The baby will arrive after 40 weeks of gestation (typically) regardless of whether you've researched every last possible health hazard or proceeded in complete ignorance.

But as any savvy person knows, to reduce unnecessary worry you should gain a full understanding of how pregnancy works and a firm grasp of basic practical concerns surrounding your pregnancy. This manual will walk you through the gestation process, which takes a bunch of cells and transforms them into a beautiful little human being who may someday ask you to babysit your grandchild.

READY OR NOT, YOU'RE PREGNANT! (pages 14–43) reviews how you got in the "family" way, discusses the early signs of pregnancy, and offers tips on selecting a healthcare provider who's a good match for you. It also explains the basics of taking care of your body while keeping fetal growth in mind, dispels myths and common worries about environmental issues that might affect your baby, and summarizes the differences of gestating one child versus multiple babies.

FIRST TRIMESTER (pages 44–73) gives a synopsis of the baby's growth from weeks 1 through 13, so you'll understand exactly why you continually feel like collapsing in a heap of exhaustion. You'll learn about what goes on at prenatal office visits, common tests offered during these weeks, what to expect from your body, and ways to minimize associated discomforts. Weight gain and food are discussed, including foods to avoid, foods to help with morning sickness, and common cravings and aversions. We'll even explain the science behind why the roast pork sandwich your colleague eats for lunch every day makes you want to hurl. Now is the time for smart exercise—for cardio and the large muscle groups and those smaller yet critical ones in the birth canal. (Hello, Kegels!) Dads-to-be will learn how to survive the hormonal roller coaster, what to say, and what not to say to their pregnant wives. She may be a wee bit touchy.

SECOND TRIMESTER (pages 74–103) describes baby's growth from weeks 14 through 26. Along the way you'll learn about highly dubious and unscientific ways to predict your baby's gender (which you will be able to determine scientifically by week 19); office visits and common tests; changes in the body; helpful tips on maternity dressing; and ways to avoid snoring like an adenoidal lumberjack. Sections will illuminate how to treat a cold or the flu, what you need to know about traveling, and how to block unwanted touching by strangers. Also provided is practical advice on signing up for birthing and breastfeeding classes and for including Dad in the baby preparations.

THIRD TRIMESTER (pages 104–135) tracks baby's growth from weeks 27 through 40. Read about office visits (which increase now), common tests during this trimester, plus changes in your body and signs of impending labor. Learn how to select a pronounceable baby name, control anxiety about labor, compile a to-do list to prepare for labor, enjoy a lovely baby shower, and pick a pediatrician, baby nurse, and daycare provider.

LAYETTE AND NURSERY (pages 136–147) relates practical tips on what baby needs immediately upon arriving at home and what supplies and equipment can wait till later. A "Just for Dads" section gives the scoop on how dads can help when choosing the major baby "hardware."

WHAT EVERY EXPECTANT DAD SHOULD KNOW (pages 148–169) shines the spotlight on Dad and what he's experiencing during this special time. Provided is information on Couvade syndrome (which may explain why he's packing on the pounds, too), which prenatal visits he is really expected to attend, and paternity leave. Also included are tips for getting mom-to-be to the hospital, how Dad can help deliver the baby if you don't make it to the hospital in time, dos and don'ts of being a birthing coach, and managing the male emotional state.

THE GRAND FINALE—HERE COMES BABY (pages 170–199) explains signals of the baby's imminent arrival, stages of labor, and essential details about the process. This chapter shares information on birthing positions, ways to avoid painkillers, what happens after baby is born, and Dad's role in this big moment. Also included are useful tips for documenting the grand arrival.

BABY ON BOARD! (pages 200–217) tells you what happens upon baby's arrival into the world and what goes on during his stay in the hospital, from cut umbilical cords and vaccines to Apgar scores and newborn screenings. We offer practical details on "rooming-in" with your baby, "kangarooing" with Dad, and other ways to maximize your hospital time before heading home. We also explain what to expect during postpartum recovery for those who delivery naturally or by a Caesarean section (C-section).

This manual is recommended for women who are considering creating a baby and for those already in the process. (Of course this book is only a general guide, and there is no substitute for discussing your individual pregnancy questions or concerns with a healthcare provider.) We consulted Dr. David Ufberg, the highly esteemed associate professor of obstetrics and gynecology at the University of Pennsylvania Health Systems. Dr. Ufberg contributed his expertise throughout the book; his personal and professional insights are featured in "Doc Talk" and "Just for Dads." Whether you breeze through pregnancy or suffer grinding discomfort from start to finish, it will all be forgotten when your little darling arrives. In fact, once the baby is born many moms confess to "pregnancy amnesia," so the next pregnancy and delivery tend to be a bit of a shock all over again. Having the proper information will help direct your energies toward the right pursuits for your health and well-being, like napping, relaxing, wholesome snacking, and shopping for all those cute baby clothes.

Congratulations, and welcome to the world of impending parenthood!

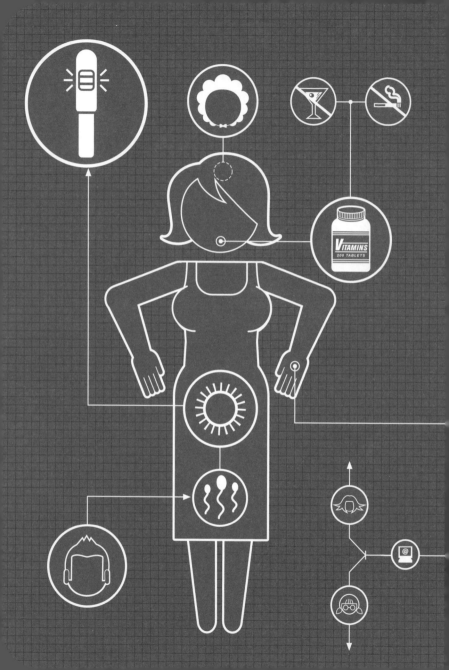

Chapter 1

Ready or Not, You're Pregnant!

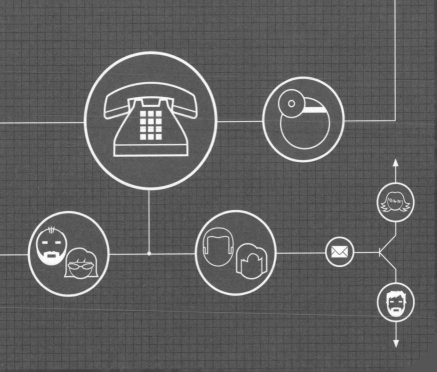

Many of us believe that the first time we have unprotected sex we'll hit that conception bull's eye, but it's rarely that easy. The average time is three to six months for sperm and egg to go out on their first date. As the saying goes: Timing is everything. The female body changes month to month. Even for the woman who has 28-day menstrual cycles like clockwork, outside factors such as stress, diet and weight changes, and recent illnesses affect how her body metabolizes hormones that affect the reproductive process.

Add to that the male factor: Sperm are completely misguided. As with many men, sperm refuse to ask for directions even as they swim blindly and with great brio down a nonovulating fallopian tube. Because of these variables, all the stars must be aligned for the boys to hit their mark.

It can be incredibly frustrating to women who are doing everything "right" only to find that it may take months before conception occurs. Remember, making the baby is the fun part—try not to turn it into a science project!

JUST FOR DADS: Many men feel as though they're put out to stud when their partner is trying to conceive. You may be having more sex than you can remember since your honeymoon, but forget about the foreplay and romance. Men, you are on that bed for one purpose alone: Make that human!

The Science of Conception

If during your high school Sex Ed class you were busy flirting with that cute classmate instead of paying attention, here is all the important information you missed.

Ovulation

Ovulation must occur to set the stage for conception. The process begins inside the woman's ovaries, where eggs ripen inside follicles, which are essentially fluid-filled sacs in which the eggs float. Around midcycle, the brain produces a surge of hormones that stimulate the egg to be released. When one egg matures, it ovulates, or breaks out of the ovary, and travels into the fallopian tube on a forward trek toward the uterus. You may be in tune enough with your own body to know when ovulation is happening. Mittelschmertz (middle pain) is the name of a constellation of abdominal symptoms that some women experience with ovulation: abdominal bloating and cramping and a dull ache on one side or the other as the egg is released. (If the egg remains unfertilized it dies and menstruation will begin, shedding the unused lining.)

Besides mittelschmertz, other signs may indicate that you are ovulating.

[1] Your cervix secretes a thinner mucus that makes it easier for sperm to travel through the vagina. Many women note the excessive mucus discharge at this time of their monthly cycle.

[2] A home-testing kit determines ovulation by measuring the amount of luteinizing hormone (LH) in your urine. When the LH rises, fertility is peaking. Because the egg is usually not released until about 24 hours after this

surge, you will know to seize the day and get thee and thy partner to the bedroom.

[3] An ovulating woman's baseline temperature will increase from a half to a whole degree after ovulation. By establishing a chart of baseline temperatures throughout several cycles, you can use a basal body temperature thermometer to track the change and identify peak fertility days.

⊕ *DOC TALK: Pregnancy care really begins months before conception. Attain your ideal pregnancy weight, lose the bad habits, eat properly, and visit your doctor or midwife three to six months before conception. Get a pap smear; complete outstanding vaccinations and blood work; and treat and manage existing medical conditions (asthma, diabetes, anxiety/depression, or hypertension). In short: Get a clean bill of health and then begin a course of folic acid or prenatal vitamins two to three months before conception.*

Fertilization

A man ejects millions of sperm at a time, but only one lucky guy gets to fertilize the egg. Sperm must reach the egg quickly once it begins its descent down the fallopian tube. The opportunity for conception dwindles as the clock ticks because the egg will die within 12–48 hours. Most sperm are lost at various points on the trip through the vagina, cervix, and uterus before reaching the appropriate fallopian tube, where still more will die.

Sperm can live up to five to seven days, so odds of conception are increased if the sperm are already in place when the ripened egg arrives on the scene.

■ If sperm and egg do meet, the remaining sperm vie for fertilization bragging rights by fighting their way through protective cell layers to get into the egg.

■ As soon as the winning sperm gets to the middle and binds to the egg, there is a breakdown and merging of the outer membranes of the sperm and egg.

■ Once fertilization has occurred, the egg undergoes the zona reaction, by which the outer egg becomes impervious to other sperm.

■ The race is over, and the remaining sperm die.

⚠ *DOC TALK: Because sperm can live five to seven days in the female genital tract, conception does not necessarily happen the same day you have sex.*

Implantation

Even though the egg is now fertilized, it still may not "take" and attach successfully to the uterine wall. As the egg and sperm do their chromosomal dance, exchanging DNA and making a complete set of 46 chromosomes, the zygote (its new name) has not yet reached its final destination in the uterus. It will take approximately three to seven days to make it to the uterine wall for implantation, at which point the zygote has transformed into a blastocyst. It is this lodging into the uterine wall that can produce light bleeding, which some women mistake for their period. Next comes the development of a placenta, which in turn begins to produce the hCG (human chorionic gonadotropin). When there's enough hCG in your system (hCG doubles every 48 hours), you will get a positive result on your urine-stick pregnancy test. And when there's enough hCG, you may also start to feel the clutching, retching feelings of morning sickness.

Hey, now you're on your way!

THE REPRODUCTIVE CYCLE

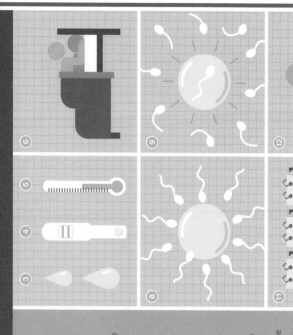

Ovulation:

1. Eggs ripen inside ovaries
2. Once ripe, eggs ovulate (break out of ovaries) and travel into fallopian tubes

Indicators of ovulation:

3. Excessive mucus discharge during monthly cycle
4. Home testing kit
5. Baseline temperature increases

Fertilization:

6. Man ejects millions of sperm. Only 1 fertilizes the egg
7. Sperm travel through the vagina, cervix, uterus, and fallopian tube to reach the egg
8. Upon meeting egg, sperm fight their way through its protective layers
9. Once fertilization has occurred, remaining sperm die

Implantation:

10. The zygote travels to the uterine wall for implantation
11. Implantation takes 3–7 days
12. Morning sickness begins

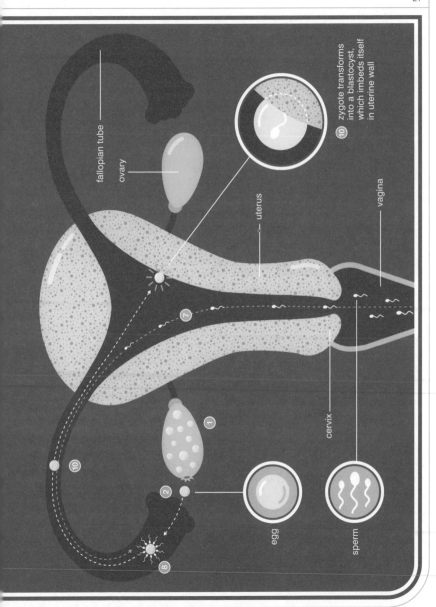

Signs You Are Not Alone

The body is not very good at keeping pregnancy a secret. Within a few weeks of conception, the mom-to-be may begin to notice that her body is definitely up to something. Some of the earliest signs of pregnancy are

Breast changes: Estrogen and progesterone hormones are changing your breasts almost within days of conception. You may feel a tingling, soreness, or heaviness in them. You may notice a darkening of the nipples and aureola.

Cramps: The growing and stretching uterus may cause cramping. This reaction is normal: a stretched muscle will respond by contracting. (Hint: Try bending over and touching your toes. That same twinge-y normal feeling in your ligaments and leg muscles is what you may feel in your uterine muscle and the ligaments that support it.) However, if you feel severe pain or experience bleeding with the cramps, contact your caregiver immediately.

Fatigue: The fatigue of first trimester pregnancy is intense. Your body is busy constructing the baby's major systems and organs, so it's no wonder you're exhausted. Rest assured, fatigue typically subsides by the end of the first 13 weeks.

Morning sickness and odor sensitivity: Expectant moms who experience nausea and vomiting, referred to as morning sickness, usually begin to feel its effects around week 5, though some begin earlier. (See page 65 for a detailed explanation and common home remedies to combat morning sickness.)

Frequent urination: The hormone progesterone is the culprit for this symptom, as is pressure on the bladder from the pregnant uterus, which sits atop it. Both the hormone and the pressure make the bladder muscles more active—sometimes when there is actually very little urine in the bladder. (If you feel a burning sensation during urination, consult your doctor since this may indicate an infection.)

Missed period or light bleeding: The bleeding occurs as the fertilized egg implants itself into the lining of your uterus. The bleeding is usually light and short-lived. But with any bleeding early in pregnancy, it is recommended that you notify your doctor, because it can sometimes be the first sign of a miscarriage or tubal pregnancy.

Hair and nail growth: Hormones have your hair and nails in overdrive. Dark hair will sprout up everywhere. Feel free to tweeze and wax. No one wants you to feel—or look—like Sasquatch during this time.

JUST FOR DADS: The early signs of pregnancy also warn Dad that he, too, is entering a confusing new landscape, one fraught with his partner's moodiness, physical changes, and sweeping fatigue. Be prepared:

- You may be rejoicing at the wonders of your partner's growing bosom, but touch them at your peril. Breast soreness is common during pregnancy. Some women even have trouble sleeping on their stomachs.
- Her bouts of utter exhaustion can be tough if you've been used to the frequent sex that led up to this state. Growing that baby is hard work, and hormones are wreaking havoc with her energy levels. Settle in! Enjoy glutting yourself on sports broadcasts or action flicks. Savor what you've always craved: total clicker control!
- If you accompany her to the toilet to comfort her when she's sick, hold her hair back gently and never, ever let her see you grimace while she barfs. That vomit-spewer is the mother of your child.

So You Think You Might Be Pregnant

There are a few ways to confirm beyond a shadow of a doubt that you are pregnant.

Home pregnancy kit: These kits check your urine for the presence of human chorionic gonadotropin (hCG) produced by the placenta. They provide the results within minutes—perhaps the most suspenseful three minutes of your life. The most sensitive types can be used as early as six to eight days after conception, or once you reach 20–25 milliliters of hCG in your system. Waiting nine to ten days past ovulation provides a more reliable result, and waiting until a missed period is even better because the time it takes for sperm and egg to meet is variable. If you happen to have a slowpoke embryo who takes his time implanting, you will have to wait longer before your body starts producing hCG. These tests may give false negatives (if the levels of hCG are too low to register) but rarely give false positives. If you get a negative result after an early test, try again in a few days and you might see it turn positive.

Office blood test: This test looks for the presence of hCG in your blood. Blood work can show a quantitative level hCG as early as one week after conception. Results may take a day or two to come back.

Ultrasound: The ultrasound, or sonogram, can reveal a pregnancy as early as five and a half weeks after conception. You will have to wait until six or seven weeks to see a heartbeat. At the eighth week, it is easy for the ultrasound to detect the baby and the heartbeat.

⚠ **EXPERT TIP:** *Use a home pregnancy kit the first time you urinate in the morning, when the highest concentration of hCG occurs.*

Dissemination of the Happy News

Holding a positive home pregnancy stick in your hand is powerful stuff. So when do you share the happy news with family members, friends, colleagues, and your other children? The question you're really asking is, When is my pregnancy a sure thing?

Timing

The old adage was to wait until you heard the baby's heartbeat at the end of the first trimester. The reason is that the human body is excellent at screening out abnormal pregnancies. Pregnancies that are not viable, whether from chromosomal abnormalities, anatomic defects, or other reasons, never reach the heartbeat stage. Now, with modern ultrasound, doctors can usually see a fetal heart beating around six to eight weeks. That means the pregnancy has passed the body's initial screening tests and is off and running. At this stage, the chance of a miscarriage drops to less than 3 percent. So, once you hit the eight-week mark, spread the news with confidence. Or just tell those people who would comfort you in case of a loss.

The timing for telling your family can be sensitive. Which grandma-to-be hears first? How do you avoid hurt feelings when one person knows and another finds out later? Keep the following suggestions in mind:

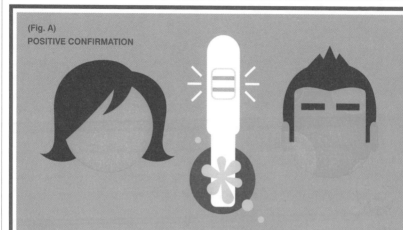

(Fig. A)
POSITIVE CONFIRMATION

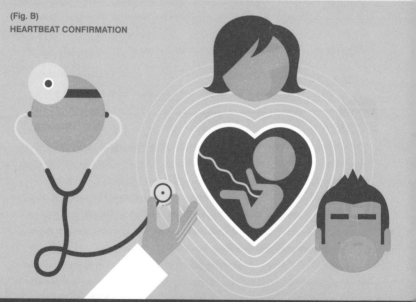

(Fig. B)
HEARTBEAT CONFIRMATION

INFORMATION DISSEMINATION: Wait until a fetal heartbeat has been

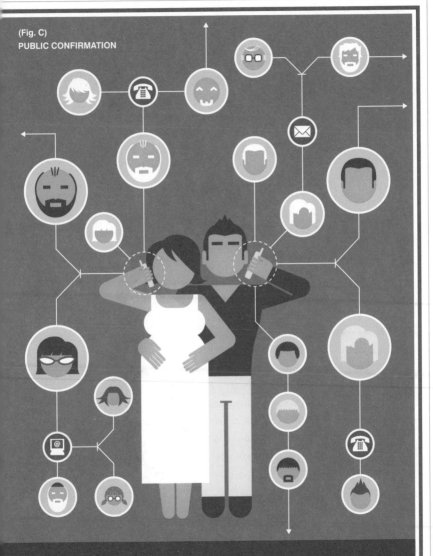

(Fig. C)
PUBLIC CONFIRMATION

detected to share the news with family members and your closest friends.

[1] A big family get-together is always a good occasion to spread the news all at once.

[2] If you are informing people one by one, avoid hurt feelings by reassuring the recipient that you wanted to share the happy news with him or her as soon as possible.

[3] If you are asked who else has been told, just stick to your story that you and your partner are trying to get the news out to everyone as soon as possible. Shift the emphasis back to the content of your message and not the order in which people were called.

[4] Your boss may also be someone who needs to know sooner rather than later, especially if he or she is a sympathetic sort and the pregnancy will affect your ability to take on assignments and complete duties. You may need time off for doctor's appointments or weathering the first trimester's rigors.

Sometimes your pregnant behaviors will give you away even if you are trying to wait. Eyebrows may be raised when those who know you well witness your sudden queasy trips to the bathroom or your abstention from a glass of wine with dinner. Feel free to lie and deny it. All will be forgiven when you do choose to tell them.

You may consider waiting to share the news for a few other reasons as well:

- Once you tell a few people, word will inevitably spread. Gossip happens, and many find it irresistible to pass along happy news.
- Your pregnant state may quickly come to feel like public property. Suddenly the contents of your womb are fair game for anyone to chat about.

Friends, acquaintances, and strangers may feel compelled to describe every pregnancy war story they know.

■ You may want an intimate circle of loved ones—sworn to secrecy until a certain agreed-upon date—to relish this special time with you.

■ You may want to keep from boring your friends and especially work colleagues. Inevitably, your pregnancy will become the most interesting topic in the world—to you—and you will likely talk and talk and talk about it once you've spilled the beans. Be aware: This can become tedious to those around you. If you wait until the end of your first trimester, you will have spared them at least three months of you prattling on about every last detail, concern, and stray thought about your changing body and growing baby.

How to Select a Caregiver

Your first task as an officially expectant mother is to select a caregiver. The person you choose will be your guide through the 40 weeks of pregnancy, teaching, reassuring, and encouraging you along the way. You must determine the setting for your child's birth (hospital, birthing center, home) and the best type of care. There are only a few options, but they can result in vastly different experiences:

Obstetrician gynecologist: With an ob-gyn, you and your child have the most complete and immediate access to all medicines, testing, equipment, and surgical procedures. Delivery will occur in a hospital.

Perinatologist or maternal-fetal medicine specialist (for high-risk pregnancies): Women choose, or are referred to, a perinatologist if they are carrying multiple fetuses, have an existing medical condition, have a history of miscarriage or difficulties with pregnancy, or develop a medical condition while pregnant. You have access to everything an obstetrician can offer as well as the additional expertise of a doctor trained to deal with complicated pregnancies. Delivery will occur in a hospital.

Family practice physician: This doctor is qualified to provide general care for women, men, and children. He has some training in obstetrics but usually will not manage a high-risk pregnancy.

Midwife: Midwifery emphasizes a personalized, holistic approach to pregnancy that does not generally employ electronic fetal monitoring, pain relief medicine, and episiotomies. Only healthy, low-risk pregnant women should opt for a midwife. There are two types:

■ A nurse-midwife has more professional training than a direct-entry midwife. She has received a degree in nursing as well as additional schooling in midwifery. Most work in hospitals, but they can deliver babies in birthing centers and homes as well.

■ A direct-entry midwife is not a licensed nurse but may have related educational degrees as a certified, licensed, or lay midwife. A direct-entry midwife typically delivers in a woman's home or sometimes at a birthing center.

What to Ask a Potential Caregiver

Ask to interview potential caregivers before making a decision about your prenatal care and delivery options.

[1] Seek recommendations from friends and family and consult magazines' "Top Docs" issues.

[2] Do a little Internet research. Check potential practitioners' references and credentials.

[3] Set up an informational interview (confirm whether you will be required to pay for the appointment).

[4] Because a caregiver may be called away to deliver a baby, ask your most important questions first. Sample questions include

☑ How many babies have you delivered?

☑ How long are your prenatal appointments?

☑ How many other doctors are in your practice and how long have they been practicing?

☑ What are the odds you will deliver my baby?

☑ What is your Caesarian-section rate (if relevant)?

☑ What are your thoughts on pain relief during labor?

☑ What hospital or birthing center are you affiliated with?

☑ Do you work with medical students in the hospital? Is it possible that a student will perform my Caesarean section or other procedures?

☑ Are you board certified?

☑ Are you comfortable working with a doula and allowing me to try nontraditional methods to ease pain and assist labor and delivery?

☑ As a midwife, what are your contingency plans if there is a medical emergency during birth for me or the baby (if relevant)?

☑ If I have to receive treatment at a hospital, how will I get there?

Besides the factual stuff, you should evaluate if the potential caregiver is a temperamental match. Does he or she "get" you? Will his or her sensibility complement your nature and neuroses and give you the stability and confidence you need during the pregnancy?

☐ Was he text messaging under his desk while you were revealing your hopes and dreams for the birth experience?

☐ Did he laugh heartily and slap his knee when you asked if a woman could remain "slim-ish" during pregnancy?

☐ Did he respond to your question about the validity of birth plans by saying, "Birth plans, shmirth plans"? Or, as you vocalized your concerns, did he immediately focus on you, leaning in while listening and nodding sympathetically?

☑ Did he give you courtesy laughs at your lame tension-defusing jokes?

☑ Did he exude the calm and wisdom of a Zen master?

☑ Did you feel like you wanted to name your child after him?

Once you've found a match, make your first prenatal appointment immediately.

Healthy Intake, Healthy Habits

The adage "Everything in moderation" was probably invented specifically for pregnant women. The occasional chocolate brownie, diet root beer, or bag of potato chips will not irreparably harm your fetus, but neither

are they the food diary entries to strive for. **When your body is building a baby, it needs all the help it can get. So feed it a balanced, sensible diet rich in grains, fruits, and vegetables and low in fat and sugar.**

Though you're already being fruitful and multiplying, for optimum baby development you will want to incorporate some important additions and subtractions into your diet.

⊕ *DOC TALK: Humans used to live in caves, and yet our species has survived and flourished. So chances are very good that in this modern age you will be able to provide all the right nutrients for your baby.*

Dietary Additions

Folic Acid: This B vitamin is found in many foods, including avocados, bananas and citrus fruit, lentils, leafy greens, and yogurt. Anyone for some lentil guacamole with a citrus smoothie chaser? Folic acid is an essential part of any diet, but it's even more critical for pregnant women. It may prevent spinal and neural-tube defects (including spina bifida and anencephaly) in the developing fetus. It is so highly regarded as a safeguard that many women begin taking supplements before conception to guarantee that their body contains enough B6 for the baby to draw upon in the critical first few weeks of development.

Prenatal Vitamins: These supplements will fill any nutritional gaps in your diet. This nutrient-rich, oversize pill (fondly referred to as a "horse pill" by countless moms-to-be) differs from the typical women's multivitamin by offering more folic acid, iron, and calcium—all critical during pregnancy. It also has less vitamin A (which, if consumed in large doses, can harm a fetus). Prenatal vitamins come in different iron dosages, so if you have a sensitive stomach, ask your caregiver for one without iron to take during the first trimester, when nausea is worst and fetal iron requirements are lowest.

⊕ **DOC TALK:** *The iron in prenatal vitamins can cause stomach problems. Take the vitamins before bedtime and you'll sleep through the worst of its nauseating effects.*

Calcium supplements: A balanced diet, along with the calcium supplement in your prenatal vitamins, will provide everything you and your baby need. Another easy form of calcium supplementation during pregnancy is calcium carbonate tablets (found in heartburn medications), which have the added benefit of settling your queasy stomach.

Omega-3 fatty acids: This supplement is a standard recommendation for pregnant women and breast-feeding moms, especially now that obstetrical guidelines urge caution and decreased fish consumption due to mercury toxicity and polychlorinated biphenyls (PCBs) levels (see page 37). Omega-3 fatty acids are linked to a baby's neurological and early visual development. Some prenatals include the long-chain polyunsaturated fatty acids found in fish or flaxseed oil. If your prenatal does not, an additional fish oil pill (obtained at any pharmacy) can be taken. Check with your doctor to get the right one for you.

Subtractions and Reductions

Illicit Drugs: Maternal drug use causes significant risk to the fetus. Depending on the drug that fetuses are exposed to, they can be born premature, with low birth weight or smaller head size; they may also suffer birth defects, postpartum neurological problems, Sudden Infant Death Syndrome (SIDS), fetal strokes, and death.

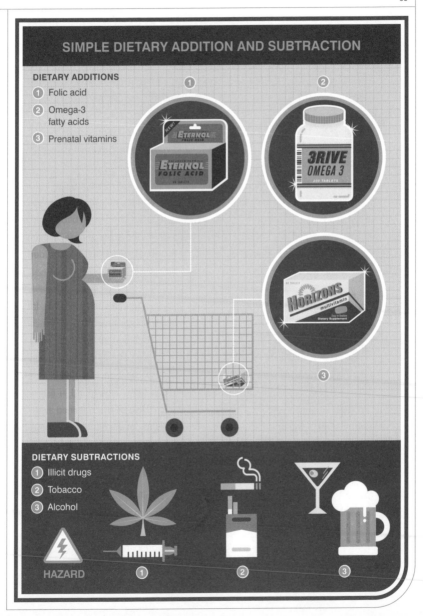

Tobacco: Smoking decreases oxygen and blood flow to the fetus. Low birth weight, stillbirth, and other gestational problems are associated with smoking when pregnant.

Alcohol: There is no safe amount of alcohol consumption during pregnancy. High consumption levels can lead to fetal alcohol syndrome (FAST), which produces birth defects (including mental retardation and heart problems). With moderation in mind, an occasional glass of wine (once a week) after the first trimester is safe.

🛨 *DOC TALK: Make sure to inform your caregiver of all your current medications, especially for conditions such as asthma, diabetes, anxiety/depression, and hypertension. Even over-the-counter medicines should be mentioned, for some of these may not be safe for your growing baby.*

Fact from Fiction: What's *Really* Dangerous to the Baby

Protecting your growing baby from dangerous toxins, chemicals, foods, and behaviors is your foremost priority. But what is safe and what isn't? Besides the obvious hazards from drugs, alcohol, and smoking, here are some clarifications:

Airport screening machines: These are safe for pregnant women. Don't let them stand between you and your last shot at a romantic getaway.

Caffeine: Cutting back on your coffee intake is not a bad idea if you're a caffeine fiend. Remember that caffeine is found in coffee, tea, soda, and chocolate. Drinking one or two caffeinated drinks daily should be fine. Keep it under 300 milligrams a day, and the fetus should remain unaffected. An 8-ounce mug of regular joe has about 95 mg, and fancier high-octane coffee may have more.

Cheese: Not all cheeses are potentially dangerous, but soft, unpasteurized cheese does pose a threat because it may carry bacteria. Avoid Brie, Stilton, Camembert, Roquefort, feta, and similar cheeses.

Chlorine: Pool chemicals are considered safe. You'll love the relief of floating in a pool, especially when you are well into the pregnancy and feel achy and bloated. Swimming is also terrific for relieving varicose veins.

Cookie dough and cake batter: Raw eggs in dough and batter may contain salmonella bacteria. Wait till those cookies and cakes are baked, then enjoy.

Electric blankets, hot tubs, and saunas: During the first trimester, a woman should keep her core temperature under 102ºF (38ºC). If your body temperature remains above that temperature for ten minutes or more, you risk damaging the fetus's neural tube and increase your chances of miscarriage. Electric blankets are unlikely to pose a problem, but if you are concerned, just use a normal blanket or enlist your partner as a source of warmth.

Fish: There is danger to the fetus's nervous system from longer-living predator fish containing high levels of methyl mercury and polychlorinated biphenyls (PCBs). Tile fish, shark, grouper, marlin, swordfish, and king mackerel should be avoided. Good news: Canned chunk-light tuna in moderation is okay.

Fumes from paints or cleaning agents: From a medical perspective, latex- or oil-based paints pose no danger. In "typical use" situations they will not cause oxygen deprivation or birth defects. Expectant mothers can paint the nursery; just make sure the room is well ventilated so that you do not become lightheaded, dizzy, or short of breath. If you do, stop immediately and get some fresh air. Try natural-based cleaning products to minimize your exposure to harsh chemical agents.

Hair dyeing, perming, relaxing, or thermal reconditioning: Chemicals from hair treatments are considered safe, but if you want to be extra cautious, wait until your first trimester has passed. Previously, dangerous formaldehyde was a common ingredient in such treatments. Simply confirm that no formaldehyde is being used. Pregnancy is no excuse for bad hair.

Hair waxing: This procedure is safe (and might be essential to combat excessive hair growth).

Herbal teas: Teas or herbs in *small quantities* have not been shown to be associated with adverse pregnancy outcomes. Some teas are even considered good for minor complaints (red raspberry and ginger for nausea; chamomile for digestion; lemon balm for anxiety and insomnia). Check with your doctor.

Horseback riding, skiing, and basketball: None of these sports is advisable while pregnant. In fact, you should avoid all activities where you could fall or get hit in the torso.

Hot dogs and lunch meat: These foods can contain the bacteria listeria. In moderation and if prepared properly, they are okay to consume. If you're craving a turkey sandwich, get fresh deli meats from a trusted supermarket or butcher. Steak tartare and other raw meat can also contain bacteria. Best to avoid.

Lead: Lead easily crosses to the placenta from the maternal bloodstream. Avoid lead paint, construction materials, and water pipes. Now is not the time to try out your amateur plumbing skills. Call a professional if repairs are needed.

Litter box: Outdoor cats can be carriers of toxoplasmosis, a disease that can infect the fetus and cause miscarriage, infant blindness, and mental retardation. Wear gloves if you must change the litter box or ask your partner or other family member to do the task. Toxoplasmosis-causing parasites are also found in soil, so remember to wash your hands thoroughly after gardening.

Microwaves: Recent models shield most radiation and thus are considered safe.

Pedicure or foot massage: Pedicures are fine—and even a necessary part of being pregnant and feeling pretty—but make sure your pedicurist uses clean equipment. Despite rumors to the contrary, there is no medical evidence that a foot massage will cause premature delivery. If you feel uncomfortable, stop the massage immediately, drink fluids, and rest. If discomfort persists, call your doctor immediately.

Pesticides: Let the weeds flourish in your yard, let the ants and moths enjoy their stay in your home and sweaters, let the Japanese beetles munch away on your rose bushes. All insecticides, herbicides, and fungicides should be avoided during pregnancy.

Reptiles: Salmonella bacteria can be passed through the feces of turtles, snakes, and lizards, so avoid their waste products and wash hands thoroughly after handling them.

Skincare: Read the ingredients label before use. Creams and lotions that contain vitamin A derivatives, especially antiaging creams, should not be used. Also Accutane, an acne treatment with vitamin A, is extremely hazardous to the fetus. Do not use. Unfortunately, now that your skin is as bad as a pizza-gobbling teenager's, you can do little about it. Time to put on that "Baby on Board" T-shirt with the big arrow pointing away from your face.

Sushi: Raw fish as well as oysters should be avoided since they can contain parasites.

Tanning machines: These emit ultraviolet radiation and are safe for the growing baby. But who needs a tan when you'll have your pregnancy "glow"?

Tattooing: The risk for infection is significant. Resist the temptation to get that "Mom" tattoo you've always wanted.

Teeth whiteners: These are safe, whether by laser or bleaching. (Whiter teeth also offer the bonus effect of drawing attention away from your growing belly, which in turn decreases the likelihood that your belly will be touched by strangers. See page 99).

Video display terminals: The rays from the monitor's electromagnetic field are considered safe.

X-rays: Low-level exposure will not be harmful.

Yoga: Yoga is a wonderful way to keep your body strong and limber and your mind clear. Practices devised specifically for the pregnant woman are ideal. However, Bikram, or Hot Yoga, practiced in a room kept at 105ºF (40ºC), is potentially dangerous, especially during the first trimester.

⊕ **DOC TALK:** *Treat yourself right and get that pedicure you've been craving. Don't worry about a foot massage sending you to the hospital early. If stimulation of the soles of the feet really caused premature contractions and early delivery, then just walking around would have ended the human race!*

Pregnant with Multiples: More, More, More

Pregnancies with multiple fetuses are much more common now than ever before, mostly due to the increased use of fertility medications by women starting families later in life.

Multiple fetuses occur either when two eggs are ovulated at the same time (and both are fertilized) to make fraternal twins or when the single zygote splits into two blastocysts, resulting in identical twins. Triplets, quadruplets, and quintuplets develop from a combination of the fraternal and identical twin scenarios, with one or multiple eggs fertilizing or when zygotes further divide to create additional blastocysts.

Multiples babies can be most easily detected by

- Ultrasound as early as week 8. If your doc is unsure, she may ask to repeat the ultrasound in two to four weeks.
- An extremely high initial hCG level.
- Above-average maternal weight gain and growth.

■ Detection of a dual heartbeat by a Doppler machine. (Be aware: Often the beating of twins' hearts is in synch and at the same rate, which can make it difficult to perceive the presence of two fetuses.)

If you're expecting multiples, your pregnancy care is generally the same for the first half of your pregnancy as it is for singleton expectant moms. Most young, healthy mothers expecting multiples have an active pregnancy without restrictions.

The main concern with twins is prematurity (the average age at delivery is 36 to 37 weeks, as opposed to 40 weeks for a single baby). If symptoms of premature labor begin, bed rest and/or hospitalization

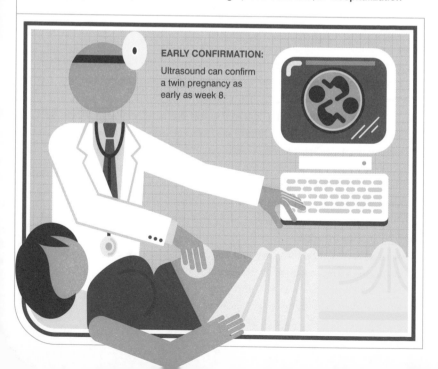

EARLY CONFIRMATION:
Ultrasound can confirm a twin pregnancy as early as week 8.

may be in order. Expectant mothers of twins are also at increased risk for gestational diabetes and preeclampsia, and moms with multiples have higher rates of Caesarean section because of increased chances of malposition of one or both twins.

With multiples, more really is more. Everything that a mom-to-be undergoes in a single-fetus pregnancy, the mother of multiples may experience exponentially:

- more hormones
- more discomfort (morning sickness, constipation, hemorrhoids, fatigue, urination, cramping, heartburn, edema, etc.)
- more weight gain
- more sleeping problems
- more strain on supporting muscles
- more testing (particularly more ultrasound scans)
- more frequent doctor's visits

Mothers of multiples also require more pampering and lots of rest. Some moms are even ordered to go on bed rest as early as week 24 to ensure ideal growth conditions and prevent preterm labor resulting from the additional gravitational stress placed on the cervix.

But don't forget the best part: You will also have more scrumptious baby after you deliver!

JUST FOR DADS: If you're having twins, get ready to start working twice as hard and be twice as understanding. And get ready to buy a diamond delivery present twice the size you were planning on.

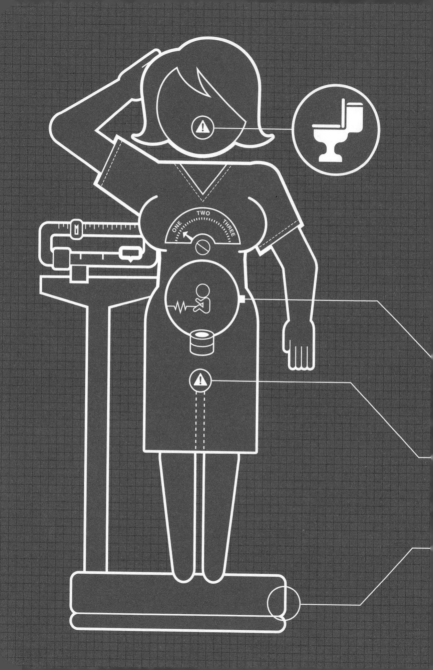

Chapter 2

First Trimester

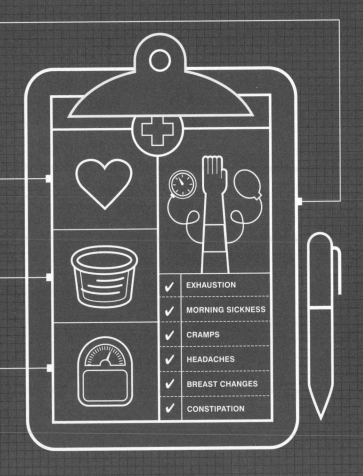

- ✓ EXHAUSTION
- ✓ MORNING SICKNESS
- ✓ CRAMPS
- ✓ HEADACHES
- ✓ BREAST CHANGES
- ✓ CONSTIPATION

Phenomenal changes occur in the first trimester, transforming the egg and sperm into a three-inch-long (7.5 cm) fetus with working organs by the end of the first 13 weeks.

Synopsis of Baby's Growth, Weeks 3–13

Here are some highlights of your little show-stopper, week by week:

Week 3: Conception. Sperm meets egg, and the zygote, transforming into a blastocyst, travels to uterus, where it attaches itself and begins growth. Placenta begins to form.

Week 4: The amniotic cavity is forming. The ectoderm (designed to develop into the brain and nervous system, skin, and hair), mesoderm (skeletal, muscular, and circulatory systems and kidneys), and endoderm (intestinal tract, lungs, and other internal organs) are growing and distinguishing themselves from one another.

Week 5: The origins of the heart form as well as the brain and skeleton.

Week 6: Brace yourself. Baby begins his most vulnerable developmental period: the embryonic state. If malformations occur, it is most often during this critical four-week period. Heart is beating. He has a brain.

Week 7: Leg buds arrive. What will be hands and arms grow longer. The origins of lungs are present and growing.

Week 8: The heart is getting more complex. Elbows and ankles arrive. The face is becoming more recognizable, with nascent eyelids, nose, tongue, and ears.

Week 9: Baby's limbs, fingers, and toes are growing longer. Reproductive organs begin to form. Baby can move!

Week 10: Baby has completed his embryonic stage and is now officially a fetus. Hooray! He even has 20 tooth buds.

Week 11: Fingernails arrive. Baby can yawn. Hair begins to grow.

Week 12: Mission completion. All major structures have been formed. You will be able to hear the heartbeat this week with a Doppler machine. Fingers and toes are no longer weblike and have separated. Baby can smile and frown. External genitalia are forming.

Week 13: Baby's intestines, which develop in the umbilical cord, are pulled into his abdominal cavity. Baby is about three inches (7.5 cm) long.

⚠️ **EXPERT TIP:** *Knowing how far along you are can be confusing. Because it is impossible to know precisely when conception occurred, doctors begin counting from the first day of your last period. So there is a two-week discrepancy between week of pregnancy and fetal week. (If you are in your 38th week of pregnancy, your baby is in her 36th week of growth.) Pregnancy is predicated on a 40-week (or 280-day) timetable (that's 38 weeks of fetal growth). Typically, babies have survived as early as 25 weeks (23 weeks of fetal growth). A baby is considered preterm if she is born before 38 weeks and postterm if she arrives after 42 weeks.*

Baby's Growth, Weeks 3–13

WEEK	STAGE			
3		✓ Sperm meets egg; forms blastocyst	✓ Blastocyst begins growth	✓ Placenta forms
4		✓ Amniotic cavity forms	✓ Ectoderm, mesoderm, and endoderm grow and distinguish themselves from one another	
5		✓ The origins form for the: ■ Heart ■ Brain ■ Skeleton		
6		EMBRYONIC STATE:	✓ Heart beats ✓ Brain is present	⚡ WARNING: Most vulnerable period begins
7		✓ The origins form for the: ■ Legs ■ Arms ■ Hands ■ Lungs		
8		✓ Heart becomes more complex	✓ Elbows and ankles form	✓ Face begins to form
9		✓ Limbs, fingers, toes grow longer	✓ Reproductive organs form	✓ Able to move
10		EMBRYONIC STATE COMPLETED: Now entering fetus stage.		✓ Tooth buds formed
11		✓ Fingernails form	✓ Hair grows	✓ Able to yawn

WEEKS

12

13

ALL MAJOR STRUCTURES FORMED!

✓ Heartbeat audible with Doppler (Fig. 1)	✓ Fingers/toes have separated (Fig. 2)	✓ External genitalia forming (Fig. 3)
✓ Able to smile/frown (Fig. 4)	✓ 3 inches (7.5 cm) long (Fig. 5)	✓ Intestines (formed in umbilical cord) move into abdominal cavity of fetus (Fig. 6)

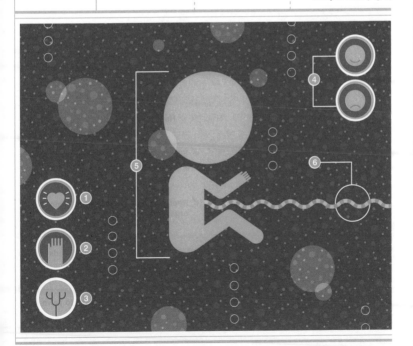

⊕ *DOC TALK: Patients often ask how we come up with 40 weeks to calculate their due date. The figure is based on population studies conducted decades ago. In the past, we did not have home pregnancy tests or early ultrasound. We had only the date of the last menstrual period and the date of delivery. After looking at the last period and delivery dates of tens of thousands of women, researchers found that 40 weeks was the most common length of pregnancy.*

Seeing Your Caregiver This Trimester

For many pregnant women, a visit to the caregiver is a much-anticipated appointment when they get to talk with someone who is just as interested in the baby as they are. You can explain every last discomfort you're suffering, get some sympathy and solutions, discuss your and the baby's weight, ask nagging questions, and receive some reassurance and encouragement. What pregnant woman doesn't love all this attention when she might be feeling just a teensy bit self-absorbed?

At your first appointment you will get even more special attention. The caregiver will set the foundation for understanding you, your medical history, and the probable course of your pregnancy. Many women bring their partner to this initial appointment. It's always helpful to have another set of ears.

Here's what to expect:

Complete medical history: Your caregiver will want to know about your health (age, diet, exercise, drinking, smoking, recreational drugs), chronic medical conditions, serious prior illnesses, surgeries, medications, allergies, gynecological history (past pregnancies, miscarriages, abortions, cysts, regularity of periods), and family history of genetic disorders.

Ultrasound: If your first appointment is in your eighth week or beyond, you will see your baby's heartbeat. (It will look like a blinking peanut.) The doctor will also be able to inform you if there are multiple fetuses (many blinking peanuts).

Physical and pelvic exam: Your height, weight, and blood pressure will be noted. The doctor will examine your whole state of wellness in addition to giving you a pelvic exam. Your caregiver may not need to repeat the pelvic exam if you have met with your doctor or midwife for a complete physical three to six months prior to this appointment (a good idea, to address any pertinent health issues, medications, or habits that could affect the critical first few weeks of pregnancy, when the anatomic structures are being formed). You might be feeling enough discomfort down there without any more poking and prodding!

Pap smear: To rule out the presence of malignant cervical cells.

Blood work: Your blood will be tested for its Rh-factor; immunity to diseases such as rubella; blood type; the presence of any sexually transmitted diseases such as HIV, syphilis, hepatitis, gonorrhea, etc.; and a complete blood count (CBC) to test for anemia.

Urine test: You will urinate into a cup, and a chemically treated paper strip will be dipped into the urine to check for the presence of protein and glucose. (If present, they might signal preeclampsia, kidney problems, or diabetes. Your doctor will confirm with further testing.)

Due date: You doctor will calculate your due date. Remember that most women do not deliver on this date, but near it. He or she will also spend time answering your or your partner's questions—nutty, reasonable, and any in between. (Will it affect my pregnancy if Fifth Disease breaks out at my older child's school? If there's an anthrax scare, will I need to be vaccinated? If I stand on my head for yoga, will my placenta tear away? If I eat peanut butter, will my baby develop an allergy to it? etc.)

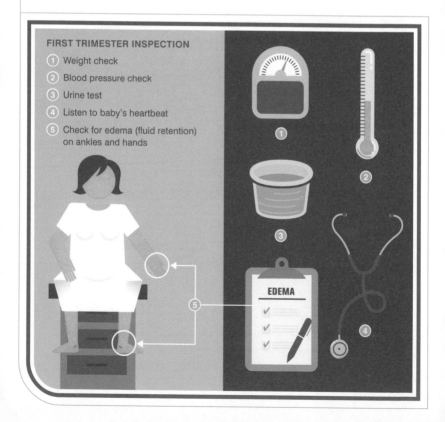

FIRST TRIMESTER INSPECTION

1. Weight check
2. Blood pressure check
3. Urine test
4. Listen to baby's heartbeat
5. Check for edema (fluid retention) on ankles and hands

In the first trimester, you will visit your caregiver only once a month (unless you're a high-risk patient). The routine is fairly standard:

- Weight check
- Blood pressure check
- Urine test
- Check for edema (fluid retention) on ankles and hands
- Listen to baby's heartbeat after the 12th week of pregnancy (probably on your second appointment) with a Doppler machine that amplifies the sound. (A baby's heart rate is between 120 and 160 beats per minute.)
- Answer questions

DOC TALK: *Many of my patients feel that they have to lock themselves in a plastic bubble and sit quietly for nine months lest they disturb the formation of organs or jar the placenta loose. Some also worry that if they are too active it can cause the baby to become entangled in its cord. I remind patients that at this point the baby is the size of a peanut, floating in a bag of fluid. Take a pea or a grape and drop it into a plastic bag full of water. Turn the bag over in your hands, and you'll see that the motion doesn't really affect the position of the pea or grape. You are pregnant, not ill, so stay active and maintain a healthy lifestyle!*

Additional Testing This Trimester

There are only a few tests you can elect to undergo in this trimester to detect chromosomal abnormalities. Some are noninvasive and some are not. Candidates for these tests include women older than 35 and those with a family history of chromosomal defects.

Chorionic villus sampling (at 9–11 weeks): The CVS test gives you many of the same results as an amniocentesis (usually done at 16–18 weeks), but it is administered significantly earlier. The screening supplies information about genetic abnormalities by extracting fetal tissue from the placenta via the cervix or through the abdomen. The rate of miscarriage as a result of performing CVS is generally quoted between 1 in 150 to 1 in 200, or less than 1 percent. The miscarriage rate has been shown to be practitioner-skill dependent, so it is imperative to find someone who is extremely experienced (such as a maternal-fetal specialist) to perform the procedure. (Amniocentesis loss rates are usually quoted as 1 in 300, but recent data have shown that it may be even less risky. The amnio loss rates seem less contingent upon the skill of the practitioner.) Results take around seven to ten days.

Nuchal translucency screening (at 11–13 weeks): This test is an ultrasound that looks at a specific area on the back of the baby's neck. A thickening of the space behind the neck has been shown to correlate highly with Down syndrome and other chromosomal abnormalities. This test is chosen by mothers who prefer not to wait until the second trimester amniocentesis to detect fetal abnormalities and by mothers who opt against the invasive and riskier chorionic villus sampling (see above).

Sequential screen (at 11–13 weeks): This screen includes the nuchal translucency ultrasound of the back of the baby's neck as well as a blood test for placental hormones PAPP-A and hCG. If these results come back with a normal reading, the patient will proceed with the quad screen (blood test) at 16 weeks (see page 85). These two results are compared and, when analyzed according to established data, offer the basis for assessing the risk level for problems. If the first part of the test is abnormal and puts the patient in a high-risk category, she is offered a CVS for confirmation of abnormalities.

Body Building: Woman at Work!

As your first trimester progresses, the early warning signs of pregnancy you first noticed will be joined by more indicators that your body is hard at work growing a baby. Remember that in the first trimester your body will build all the baby's major structures and then some, so it's easy to see why the following side effects are common:

Exhaustion: In the first trimester fatigue can be so staggering that it is almost liberating: Resistance is futile. When it hits, you can't make efforts to keep going because you are already soundly asleep. It is different than the nagging, creeping weariness that descends in the final trimester. So steal as many naps as you can throughout the day. Go to bed early and exercise to get a jolt of energy. Anemic bodies are tired bodies, so don't forget to take your prenatal vitamins to prevent an iron deficiency. Your body is producing more blood, so your iron levels can dip, especially if you are vomiting.

Morning sickness: This lovely side effect—caused by hormones, stress, odor sensitivity, sluggish digestion—usually phases out by the end of this trimester. (See page 65 for greater detail and some popular curatives.)

Cramps: Your uterus and the ligaments that support it are growing and stretching—most uncomfortably at times.

Headaches: Hormones can generate headaches, which are often worse in the first trimester. Acetaminophen or ibuprofen can be used for relief. Dehydration can also contribute to headaches, so make sure you drink enough fluids. Early pregnancy can strongly resemble a hangover for about 12 weeks, but without all the fun the night before.

Urination: Hormones are also making your bladder more active, and pressure from the baby, who is sitting atop, is tricking your bladder into thinking it needs to be emptied more frequently. Your kidneys will also have extra urine because they are filtering the significantly increased amount of blood your body is producing. All the water you're drinking to make your headaches and constipation go away—and keep dehydration at bay if you're struggling with morning sickness—will also add up to more fluid to flush out of your system.

Breast changes: In addition to tenderness and darkening of the aureolas, you may notice increasing networks of blue veins on your breasts as blood supply in them is increasing. Your breasts are beginning preparations to supply breast milk. They will grow steadily throughout this trimester. Some larger-breasted women may resort to a good support bra for more comfortable sleeping. Breast tenderness and enlargement are normal, and as hormones stabilize around 10–12 weeks the soreness will usually pass. (Or you may just forget about it as you move on to some other bodily symptom that bugs you more.)

Constipation: Hormones are making your intestinal system sluggish so that you can absorb every last nutrient from the food you take in. Also, as your uterus grows, it smushes the intestines and rectum, leading to bloating, constipation, gas, and heartburn. Water and a fiber-rich diet can help speed the bowels along. Natural laxatives such as dried fruits and prune juice offer relief, too. In the most severe cases, ask your doctor to recommend a stool softener and motility agents. Both are safe.

Varicose veins and hemorrhoids: Just one more of the many pleasures of pregnancy. Some women will have large hemorrhoids that persist for weeks or even months. When veins cannot transport blood back to the heart efficiently, the blood can accumulate at certain locations, creating varicose veins (in the legs and vagina) and hemorrhoids (in the rectum). The weight gain women experience in pregnancy exacerbates this condition, along with the pressure on veins from the growing uterus. What you can do:

■ Alleviate these effects by putting up your legs as often as you can to take the weight off the uterus and pelvic veins and to improve circulation.

■ Exercise to get the blood chugging around your system. Swimming helps.

■ To pamper your hemorrhoids, give them a 20-minute sitz bath. (Sitz baths are also recommended for episiotomy recovery, so chances are you'll find more than one occasion for use.)

■ Ask your doctor for a prescription for a mild steroid to calm hemorrhoids.

■ Use witch hazel pads to alleviate hemorrhoid pain.

■ Increase your intake of fiber and water to stimulate the colon for less straining while moving bowels. Straining is a no-no and will only make those hemorrhoids grow!

Dizziness and heart palpitations: As your body experiences significant changes in its circulatory system, your blood volume will increase by half, making your heart work that much harder. Much of your blood flow is directed to your uterus, which can leave you feeling lightheaded. Additionally, the baby can press on key return veins, which will produce blood pressure drops. Keep your blood-sugar levels and hydration steady to prevent distress. Heart palpitations are worse during hot summer months. It is estimated that the normal regular heart rate increases about 20 beats per minute during pregnancy. If you have a resting heart rate of 80, it will now be 90 to 100. With even minimal exertion that rate can jump to 110 or 120 beats a minute. This increase may worry some patients.

- Shift your position or sit down if you feel faint.
- Lie down on your left side if your heart is racing or you have shortness of breath. The symptoms should pass quickly.
- Stand up slowly to prevent getting "stars" in front of your eyes.

Excess saliva (pytalism): Those lucky women who experience morning sickness are more likely to experience extra spit as well. Sucking on anything citrus is a popular home remedy to help reduce the overproduction of saliva.

Mood swings: Is pregnancy like PMS on steroids? For some. The combination of hormones and the stress that can arise from contemplating how your life will soon change can result in serious irritability and weepiness. Rest assured that this territory is familiar for all pregnant women. Most seasoned moms have a favorite recollection of tearing up at some schmaltzy movie, commercial, or greeting card that would have produced eye-rolling before pregnancy. Mood swings should level out at the end of this trimester before resurfacing when birth is imminent. Consult your doctor if your emotions are too intense to manage or you experience signs of depression.

Skin changes: With surging pregnancy hormones, you may feel like it's puberty all over again. Most women experience some breakouts. Clean your face with a gentle soap and water and hang in there. Do not use acne medicines or antiwrinkle creams, which may contain ingredients linked to fetal deformities.

⚠️ **EXPERT TIP:** *Take a deep breath and . . . release. You may experience times of considerable irritability while pregnant. See it for what it is: normal pregnant behavior. You are tired, physically uncomfortable, and possibly anxious. Crabbiness is normal—just try to keep the collateral damage to a minimum. And try some smart coping strategies: reduce your intake of caffeine, sugar, and salt; take a nap; exercise; or change your focus with a book, movie, or other diversion that engages your attention. Being alone until you can get yourself together is a good coping strategy for some women, whereas others may need the support of sympathetic friends and family who can make them laugh.*

Healthy Habits

The real scoop on weight gain can be a bit deflating: Eating for two is a myth. You need to add only up to 300 calories a day to your diet to sustain healthy fetal growth (more if you have multiples). As your pregnancy progresses and your physical activity diminishes, you may not even need to consume many additional calories since you won't be burning what you used to.

Yet weight gain is a strong sign of healthy growth, and caloric restrictions can lead to underweight and even premature babies. Dieting is dangerous to the fetus and deprives the baby of essential vitamins and minerals. The old adage—nine months to put on, nine months to take off—is one to embrace to ease your weight-gain woe. Just focus on consuming a well-balanced diet with lots of fruits and vegetables, plenty of protein, and moderate carbs.

Pregnancy by the Numbers

- underweight women should gain 28–40 pounds (13–18 kg)
- normal weight women should gain 25–35 pounds (11–16 kg)
- overweight women should gain 15–25 pounds (7–11 kg)
- women carrying twins should gain 35–45 pounds (16–20 kg)

But everyone is different. Most women will gain an average of 5–15 pounds (2–7 kg) in the first half of pregnancy and then approximately 1 pound (.5 kg) per week from 20 weeks until full term. The first trimester reveals a lot of fluctuation from the average because of the profound effect of hormones and appetite. Many women will stay the same weight or even lose some weight because of nausea, lack of appetite, and vomiting. As long as you stay well hydrated and the baby is growing appropriately, be reassured that the baby will take what she needs and weight gain will come in time.

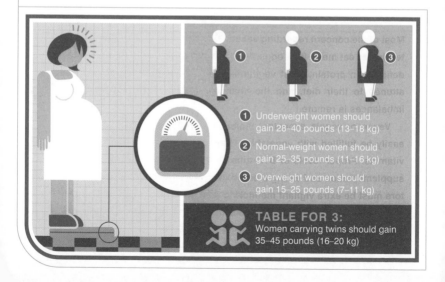

1. Underweight women should gain 28–40 pounds (13–18 kg)
2. Normal-weight women should gain 25–35 pounds (11–16 kg)
3. Overweight women should gain 15–25 pounds (7–11 kg)

TABLE FOR 3:
Women carrying twins should gain 35–45 pounds (16–20 kg)

If your weight gain is excessive, your doctor may suggest screenings for possible underlying hormonal disorders, diabetes, and thyroid disease. Nature is very good at protecting its investment, so even moms with chronic disease can usually expect a good outcome.

⊕ *DOC TALK: Moms-to-be will often report that they are eating and exercising the same amount but are still gaining weight. I remind them that much of this weight gain is fluid. During pregnancy the body is a sponge. Because of the propensity to absorb fluid, patients will be sensitive to foods high in sodium. If you eat Chinese food or pizza late in pregnancy, you may see remarkable weight shifts. Usually these shifts are simply due to the body equilibrating.*

Going Green? Tips for Vegetarian and Vegan Pregnancies

Most of the concern regarding vegetarian or vegan moms-to-be (the latter do not eat meat, fish, eggs, fowl, or dairy) is that they may become deficient in protein. Most vegetarians and vegans are already highly attuned to their diet, and the chance of significant deficiencies or imbalances is remote.

Vegan or veggie expectant moms' vitamin and mineral needs can easily be fulfilled with vegetables, fruits, fortified foods, and prenatal vitamins. Proper levels of B12, zinc, and iron can be attained through supplementation and eating a broad, well-balanced diet. However, doctors must be extra vigilant monitoring fetal growth for these moms and will administer more frequent tests to make sure there are no electrolyte imbalances.

Some good nonanimal protein sources for expectant moms include:

■ Soy products (soy milk, tofu, tempeh, edamame)

■ Legumes such as lentils, nuts, seeds, beans (For convenience try peanut butter, hummus, chili, and baked beans. For ultimate convenience grab a readymade protein shake.)

■ Wheat germ (Get a jar and just sprinkle it over hot or cold cereal and into baked goodies, salads, yogurt, or casseroles.)

■ Remember to combine proteins with wholegrain products (whole wheat breads, brown rice, and the like) for a complete complement of amino acids.

Food Cravings

Sometimes it seems as though your baby is the fussiest customer at the uterus café, one who won't stop making bizarre menu requests. The classic craving is pickles and ice cream. Some women crave chocolate, spicy red sauce on pasta, or grapefruit. Tune in to what your baby and your body are hungering for. Spicy food could be a plea for more salt in response to increasing blood volume. Grapefruit could be a call for more vitamin C. Hormones are linked to cravings, too, which can be most intense in the first trimester.

You know you're having a craving if you must have one of these foods—and lots of it—right away:

■ chocolate chip cookies
■ chocolate milk
■ pickles
■ oranges and lemons
■ cherries, strawberries
■ peanut butter
■ spinach

■ beef jerky
■ cottage cheese
■ almonds
■ milkshakes
■ fresh-baked bread
■ French fries

FOOD CRAVINGS: Tune into what your body and baby are hungering for.

YOU MAY EXPERIENCE INTENSE CRAVINGS FOR:

1. Grapefruit, lemons, oranges
2. Strawberries, cherries
3. Almonds
4. Chocolate
5. Spicy red sauce on pasta
6. French fries
7. Chocolate chip cookies
8. Milkshakes

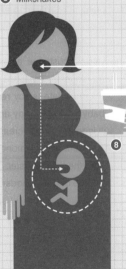

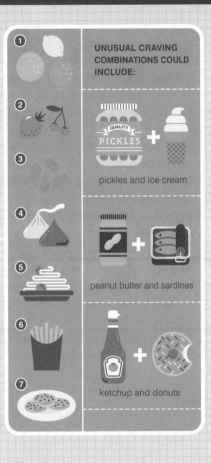

UNUSUAL CRAVING COMBINATIONS COULD INCLUDE:

QUALITY PICKLES +

pickles and ice cream

+

peanut butter and sardines

+

ketchup and donuts

⚠ CAUTION: Beware of pica (dangerous non-food cravings for clay, chalk, laundry starch, etc.)

⚠ **Caution:** *Pica, an extreme and dangerous form of nonfood cravings, compels women to eat substances that can be fatal to the fetus (including clay, laundry starch, and chalk). Pica has been associated with iron deficiencies. Notify your doctor at once if you suspect you have pica.*

Morning Sickness

Morning sickness is not just a pregnant woman's early morning wake-up call. The nausea and vomiting can strike any time of day. For women who experience morning sickness, it is worst during the first trimester. Some unlucky women continue to experience nausea and vomiting into the second; and a rare few have it throughout gestation. (The most extreme form is called hyperemesis gravidarum and can lead to hospitalization to prevent dehydration, weight loss, and other issues. Nutritional supplementation can be required for the most severe and prolonged cases.)

Surging hormones (progesterone and human chorionic gonadotropin, or hCG) are the suspected culprits behind morning sickness, though stress, fatigue, odor sensitivity, fluctuating blood-sugar levels, and sudden motion on an empty stomach are other contributing factors. Though unpleasant, morning sickness is often regarded as a positive sign that the placenta is busy and working nicely. Progesterone also contributes to queasiness by slowing the speed at which the stomach empties.

Babies are great parasites and will take what they need from the mom, even when maternal food intake is minimal. The only truly concerning aspect of morning sickness is the potential for dehydration. Contact your doctor if you cannot keep down fluids for 24 hours or if you feel persistently lightheaded and dizzy (both signs of dehydration).

There are medicines to inhibit nausea and vomiting for the extreme cases, but most moms prefer to manage their symptoms with home remedies.

Ginger: Moms swear by anything gingery (cookies, hard candies, lollipops, ginger tea, ginger ale, raw ginger).

Crackers, toast, pretzels, saltines: Bland carbs are easy to digest. Keep some by your bedside table and have a few before starting the day.

Vitamin B6: Consume 25 mg three times a day. This popular supplement might be filling in nutritional gaps that help remedy the queasies.

Cola or cola syrup: This old standby helps combat nausea.

Lemon: Tart, sour tastes and smells help some sufferers.

Herbal teas (chamomile, peppermint, or raspberry leaf): Some herb teas aid digestion, which can ameliorate nausea.

Accupressure wristbands: The same ones used for sea sickness.

⊕ *DOC TALK: Nausea and morning sickness are both normal and potentially protective to mom and baby. In fact, morning sickness is believed to be an evolutionary protection system: Many of the food aversions in the first trimester are to red meat, chicken, fish and seafood, and dairy products. These foods can spoil easily and, if not cooked properly, lead to food poisoning, with potentially harmful bacteria traveling to the developing fetus. So all that vomiting is a good thing. Really.*

Getting Physical

Embracing your inner couch potato is not a wise strategy. Sure, you may feel tired and awkward, but exercise can help your body in so many ways. The benefits are worth putting down that bag of chips and celebrity gossip magazine and hauling yourself off the couch. (Check with your doctor to make sure you are cleared for exercise.) Consider some of the benefits:

- Exercising and fresh air may take your thoughts off morning sickness.
- Refocusing your mind from your body to the great big world around you will help alleviate moodiness.
- Pumping blood helps take pressure off varicose veins and hemorrhoids.
- Increasing motility in your colon will relieve constipation and gas.
- Stretching and moving your legs will decrease the likelihood of leg cramps.
- Exercising produces endorphins that can stop headaches in their tracks and counteract fatigue.
- Developing muscle strength and stamina reportedly shortens the duration of labor.

Before hitting the jogging trails or stationary bike, remember:

[1] You may need a more substantial exercise bra if your breasts are tender and need support.

[2] You will need to keep well hydrated.

[3] If you feel overexerted, faint, or dizzy, stop immediately and sit down until you recover.

[4] Your mantra should be: Listen to your body. If you were a 10K-a-day runner, you may need to reevaluate what your body is capable of as pregnancy progresses. Continue to do so as the weeks pass.

[5] As your ligaments loosen and your weight increases, your balance may become less reliable. Bear that in mind as you choose your activities.

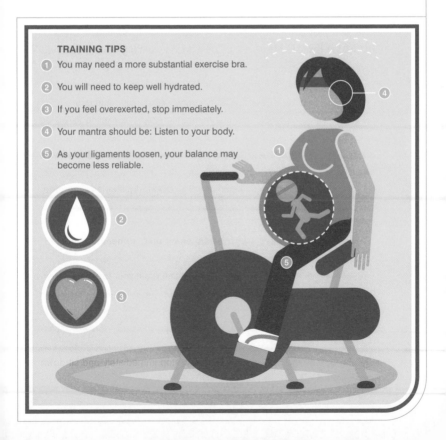

TRAINING TIPS

1. You may need a more substantial exercise bra.
2. You will need to keep well hydrated.
3. If you feel overexerted, stop immediately.
4. Your mantra should be: Listen to your body.
5. As your ligaments loosen, your balance may become less reliable.

How Hot Is Too Hot?

One concern expressed by women who want a workout is that they may put the fetus at risk by increasing their heart rate and body temperature. A wise guideline is that you should be able to maintain a conversation during exercise. Once you begin panting or gasping for breath, your body is too challenged. Another recommendation is to keep the heart rate between 130 and 140 beats per minute, though athletes may challenge themselves with greater intensity.

Beneficial exercise

Most women should feel free to continue prepregnancy exercises and taper exertion levels as the trimesters pass.

Walking and swimming are blue-ribbon activities: loss of balance is rare, you are unlikely to get poked in the stomach, and you can go at your own pace. Water helps relieve pressure on the pelvis and back and loosens muscles in the upper back. It also improves circulation in the lower extremities. Yoga also provides a good, gentle workout for pregnant women, though you will not be able to do certain poses after your uterus reaches a certain size. Join a pregnancy yoga class to learn the basic poses recommended for each trimester.

Biking is recommended, but you may want to switch to a stationary bike as the pregnancy progresses to avoid risking loss of balance.

All women, whether fit or flabby, should embrace the Kegel. This exercise, named for obstetrician-gynecologist Dr. Arnold Kegel, works to strengthen the muscles in the pelvic floor. Not only will it help your vagina push out the baby, it will also strengthen muscles to prevent urinary leakage during and after giving birth and speed postpartum recovery. Kegeling has been linked to greater satisfaction during intercourse—for both participants.

[1] Identify the muscles by attempting to stop urine flow while peeing. If you can do that, then you know you've located the correct muscles.

[2] Squeeze the muscles together.

[3] Hold for 15 seconds.

[4] Release.

[5] Complete three sets of 15 squeezes at a time.

⚠ *EXPERT TIP: Do your sets after each meal, and you'll get in the habit of working out those muscles.*

Sex After Conception

Sexual drive after conception can be unpredictable: Some women feel fat and yucky, and their sex drive dries up; others feel nearly rapacious in their sexual needs; still others are on a roller coaster of high and low. Some men feel uneasy about having relations when their child-to-be is present or even that penetration will hurt the fetus or mother. (It won't.)

Whatever you and your partner are feeling, you are not alone. Simply note that sexual relations should not pose a risk to your growing baby, unless you are a high-risk patient. Check with your doctor.

A pregnant woman's changing body, however, does come with certain logistical restrictions. You may be less comfortable lying on your back after the first trimester because of the pressure on your veins. If you feel faint, shift your weight. You don't want to be rushed to the emergency room in your sexy maternity lingerie. Opt for other positions that work for both partners.

COITUS INTERRUPTUS: Sexual relations can continue after conception,

SHE MAY BE CONCERNED WITH:

1 Weight she's gained

but sex drive may dry up for some couples due to various concerns.

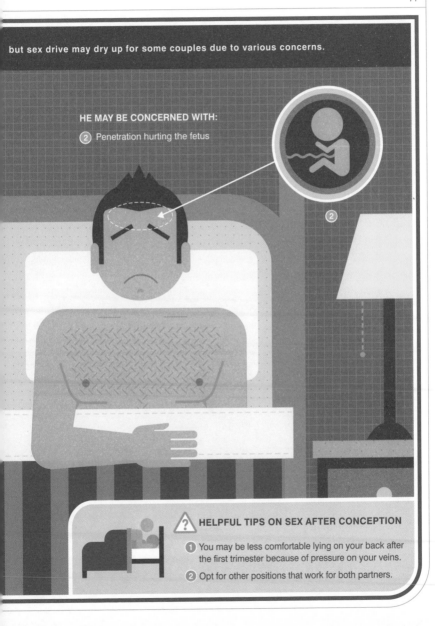

HE MAY BE CONCERNED WITH:

② Penetration hurting the fetus

HELPFUL TIPS ON SEX AFTER CONCEPTION

① You may be less comfortable lying on your back after the first trimester because of pressure on your veins.

② Opt for other positions that work for both partners.

Size of Fetus as Depicted in Oft-Repeated Fruit Analogies

Are you or your partner having a hard time conceptualizing just how big your growing baby is? Try using this handy fruit analogy chart. The next time you walk around the produce section of your supermarket, just ask your partner to pick up that small watermelon and imagine carrying it around 24/7. Don't look for too much sympathy if you're only eight weeks pregnant. That little grape is nothing to gripe about.

- 8 weeks: grape
- 12 weeks: plum
- 16 weeks: orange
- 20 weeks: grapefruit
- 28 weeks: cantaloupe
- 36 weeks: small watermelon

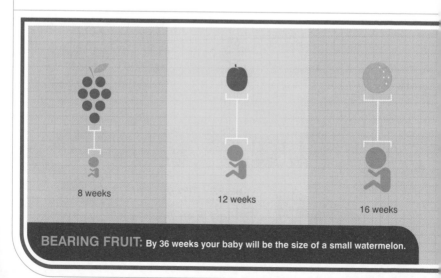

8 weeks

12 weeks

16 weeks

BEARING FRUIT: By 36 weeks your baby will be the size of a small watermelon.

⚠ **JUST FOR DADS:** *Hang on, because the roller coaster is really going now. You may have trouble understanding your partner's mental and physical changes. Try not to feed the fire and react emotionally when she seems irrational. Stay rested and count to one thousand. It will pass. Just remember your mantra: "I am wrong, and I'm sorry." Also remember that this experience is good parenting training. You may come home after a long day at work and walk into a maelstrom. These storms are a daily part of parenting and are completely unpredictable. Stay rested and find your happy place. Think big picture, and don't be afraid to keep your own daily log of events. I guarantee that at your child's first birthday, you and your partner will read the entries and have a good laugh. (She may even feel so apologetic that you'll get some extra attention!)*

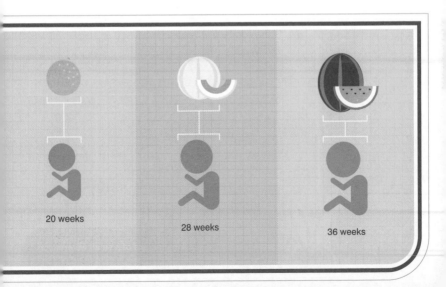

20 weeks

28 weeks

36 weeks

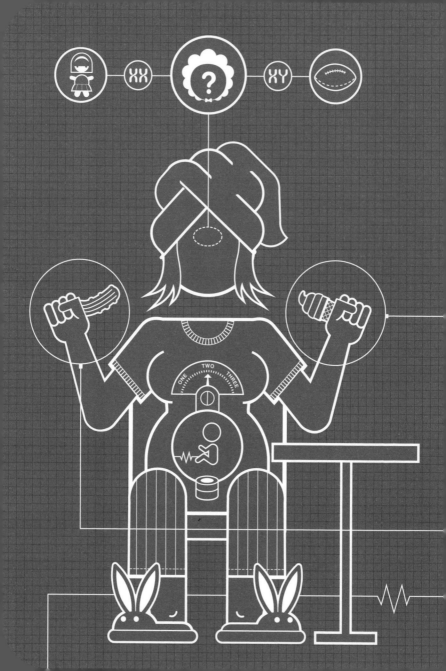

Chapter 3

Second Trimester

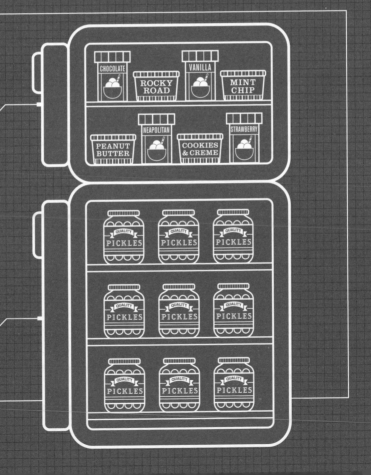

If there is a trimester to love, this is the one: You're showing, but you've not yet become ungainly. Your morning sickness and headaches should have passed. Your all-consuming fatigue has diminished—though you still love a good nap. Sleeping and digestion difficulties do not yet head up your list of woes (as they will toward the end of pregnancy). In a sense, you have hit cruising speed for the next three months before your body will have to brace itself for "landing."

Synopsis of Baby's Growth, Weeks 14–26

Here are some highlights of your little peanut week by week in this trimester:

Week 14: Baby is beginning to replicate lung function by "breathing." This inflow and outflow of amniotic fluid helps the development of lung tissue and respiratory muscles. They will need to be strong when the baby breathes on her own after birth. Until then, she's getting her oxygen from mom's blood, which travels through the umbilical cord.

Week 15: Baby is beginning to grow fine hair on her body, called lanugo. Baby can suck her thumb.

Week 16: External genitalia are complete.

Week 17: Baby is starting to get fat layers. She can hear.

Week 18: Baby is quite active in the uterus by this point.

Week 19: Meconium is being generated in the bowels. This substance will eventually be baby's first poop. (Awww.)

Week 20: You are halfway to the end of your pregnancy.

Week 21: She has her own sleep schedule by now.

Week 22: Baby has fingerprints. Most women can feel baby move by this week, even those who have the placenta on the anterior wall of the uterus (see "Doc Talk" below).

Week 23: Baby is drinking and processing her amniotic fluid.

Week 24: Most practitioners will declare that baby has reached viability. He or she can now potentially survive outside the womb.

Week 25: Fetal movements become more distinct and regular, usually most intensely after meals and before bedtime.

Week 26: Baby's eyes are complete. Her lungs are making surfactant, which prevents stickiness in the lungs' structures.

✚ *DOC TALK: By week 22, almost all women will feel their baby move. Some will feel kicking earlier, and some later. The variation can be attributed to the location of the placenta. If the placenta is on the back wall of the uterus (or the "posterior" position), the baby will be closer to the nerves of the anterior abdominal wall, and the mom can feel movement as early as week 16. Conversely, if the placenta is located on the anterior, or front, wall, it acts as a sensation dampener, and the movements of the fetus are not*

Baby's Growth, Weeks 14–26

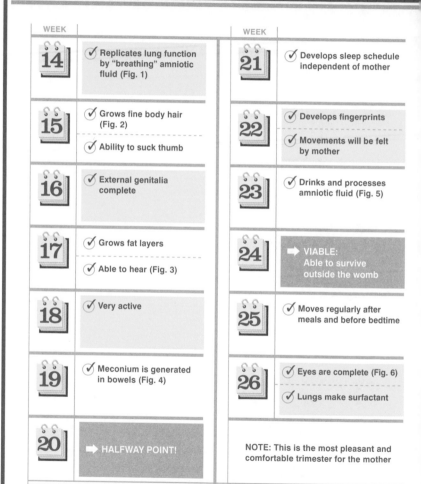

WEEK

14 ✓ Replicates lung function by "breathing" amniotic fluid (Fig. 1)

15 ✓ Grows fine body hair (Fig. 2)

✓ Ability to suck thumb

16 ✓ External genitalia complete

17 ✓ Grows fat layers

✓ Able to hear (Fig. 3)

18 ✓ Very active

19 ✓ Meconium is generated in bowels (Fig. 4)

20 ➡ HALFWAY POINT!

WEEK

21 ✓ Develops sleep schedule independent of mother

22 ✓ Develops fingerprints

✓ Movements will be felt by mother

23 ✓ Drinks and processes amniotic fluid (Fig. 5)

24 ➡ VIABLE: Able to survive outside the womb

25 ✓ Moves regularly after meals and before bedtime

26 ✓ Eyes are complete (Fig. 6)

✓ Lungs make surfactant

NOTE: This is the most pleasant and comfortable trimester for the mother

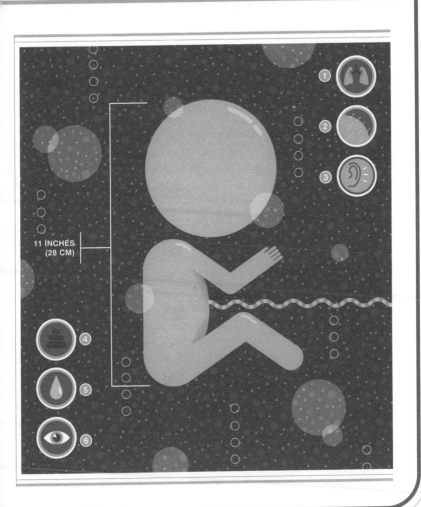

11 INCHES
(28 CM)

strong enough to register until later, when the baby is larger. Women with anterior placement usually luck out in the sleep department since they aren't as hassled by the baby's kicking and jabbing.

Step Right Up and Try Your Luck: Predicting Baby's Sex

People just love to speculate on whether you are having a boy or a girl. Old ladies, in particular, feel as though they have cornered the market on guessing a baby's sex. Here are some of the unreliable strategies they employ. (Remember, there's no medical basis for any of these.)

■ Are you carrying high or low? It's a girl if it's high, a boy if it's low.

■ Craving sour food means it's a boy, and craving sweet things means it's a girl.

■ If your baby's heartbeat is more than 150 beats per minute, it's a girl; if it's below, it's a boy.

■ Bad skin means that you're having a girl. (A girl will "steal her mother's looks.")

■ If your nose widens, it's a boy. (So much for girls stealing mom's looks.)

■ If someone hangs a wedding ring on a string over your belly and it moves in a circular motion, you are having a boy; a back and forth motion indicates you are having a girl.

■ If your belly looks like a beach ball, it's a boy; if it looks like a watermelon, it's a girl.

■ If you have bad morning sickness, it's a girl.

■ If you have cold feet (more than what you experienced prepregnancy), you're having a boy.

■ If Dad is gaining weight during your pregnancy, it's a boy.

Seeing Your Caregiver: What Goes on Behind Those Closed Doors

During your second trimester, you will still visit your caregiver once a month (unless you are a high-risk patient, and then you will go more frequently). The routine, as in the first trimester, is fairly standard. In addition to answering questions about symptoms you're experiencing, your caregiver will:

■ Check your weight

■ Check your blood pressure

■ Check your urine for glucose, protein, and blood. High sugar levels could mean diabetes; protein could suggest that the kidneys are not working properly and may indicate preeclampsia; blood might suggest infection or kidney stones.

■ Check for edema (fluid retention) on ankles and hands. Excessive swelling could suggest preeclampsia.

■ Listen to baby's heartbeat

■ Check location of fundus (top of the uterus) to monitor fetal growth

All Systems Go? Testing This Trimester

You're feeling better now—what's wrong?

That's the way a lot of women feel this trimester, when nausea and fatigue begin to wane. You don't really show much yet and may not feel the baby moving that much. That gives you a lot more free time to think, "Gee, I'm not racing for my vomit bag so much; let me use this time to dwell on the fact that I don't think my baby has kicked in more than an hour."

It's not uncommon for your doctor to get a phone message like: "Feeling great, energy is back, but I'm really worried that something is wrong. Call me back ASAP!" So although all these second trimester tests may be giving you the yips, they are actually meant to reassure you and your partner that your baby is developing normally. (And if the tests do come back indicating something abnormal, you now have the information to do something about it or simply educate yourself.)

It's pretty hard to top the surreal thrill of witnessing your baby swim around the womb on an ultrasound scan. Yet watching the television screen also produces a curiously detached feeling: "Hmm . . . fascinating," until you remember, "Hey, that's going on *inside* me!"

Amniocentesis (possible at weeks 15 through 18, but usually at 16 weeks): Not all women have this test performed, but it is an option for women older than 35 (who have increased risk for fetal malformations), women carrying multiples, or women with a family history of birth defects.

How it's done:

[1] The abdomen is sterilized and the needle is inserted into the amniotic sac. No anesthetic is used because there are relatively few nerve fibers in the lower abdomen. Just pinch the skin around your belly button as hard as you can. See? Not so bad.

[2] The doctor uses an ultrasound machine to guide the needle's placement, avoiding placenta and baby.

[3] Amniotic fluid is extracted.

[4] The fetal cells are isolated from the amniotic fluid and cultured in a lab until the DNA can be analyzed to ensure that the chromosomal count is correct. There should be 46 matching chromosomes and two sex chromosomes (either XX or XY). Sometimes specific genetic diseases can be tested for, including cystic fibrosis or sickle cell disease.

[5] Results are received in about ten days.

Bonus points: Baby's sex can also be confirmed at this time, with 100 percent accuracy—that is, if you want to know.

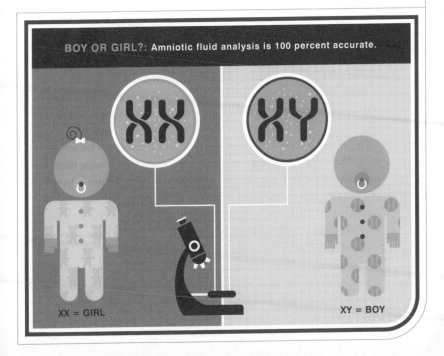

BOY OR GIRL?: Amniotic fluid analysis is 100 percent accurate.

XX = GIRL

XY = BOY

Ultrasound (at 21–22 weeks): This extremely thorough examination evaluates the anatomy of the fetus in detail (not just counting fingers and toes) and screens for problems in the internal organs, bony structures, placenta, and umbilical cord. It is also referred to as a Level 2 ultrasound or anatomy scan. You can also determine the baby's sex at this session (if you choose to learn it and baby cooperates).

⚲ **EXPERT TIP:** *If you do not want to know your baby's sex, tell the technician as soon as he or she walks in the exam room. Then ask the tech to let the doctor know your wishes when the two of them have their hallway pow-wow over the findings. Otherwise the doc may unwittingly spill the beans.*

♂ **JUST FOR DADS:** *Don't miss the second trimester anatomy scan. Seeing the baby move around your partner's womb will make you realize what she's been acutely aware of from Day One: You're pregnant! There's nothing like seeing a tiny little skeletal hand waving back at you from the screen, or sucking her tiny thumb, or draping her arm over her head, to make you suddenly grow up and realize you're the one who will be her source of comfort, wisdom, and love.*

Glucose tolerance test (at 25–28 weeks): How sweet it is. This screening for gestational diabetes is given at the close of your second trimester or beginning of the third. You will drink what tastes like sweet soda (50 grams of glucose solution) and have your blood drawn one hour later. If your results return positive for gestational diabetes, you will take a diagnostic three-hour test to confirm the results.

Most women who have gestational diabetes are initially placed on a no-sweets/low-carbohydrate diet and their sugars are monitored. No sneaking in powdered donuts—not even the mini ones! If the sugars remain persistently high, medications such as insulin may be required to keep them in a normal range.

⚠ *DOC TALK: In a perfect world, everyone would have a three-hour glucose test because it gives a much clearer picture of glucose metabolism in pregnant women over a long period. But this test is a huge pain in the rear. Ask a pregnant woman not to eat for an 8- to 12-hour period and you've got a fight on your hands. What studies have found is that you can easily screen out a large percentage of low-risk women by doing the nonfasting one-hour glucose test.*

Not at Your Local Multiplex: AFP, Triple, and Quad Screenings

None of the following screenings that look for the possibility of Down syndrome and spina bifida is diagnostic. If the screening tests come back with certain results, an amniocentesis or high-level ultrasound will be recommended for confirmation. The quad screen is the most sensitive and commonly ordered test, though you should double-check with your doctor so you know which test you are taking and why.

Alpha-fetaprotein testing (at 16–18 weeks): The baby produces alpha-fetaprotein (AFP), which crosses into your bloodstream. This test is a simple blood draw. Elevated levels of AFP might indicate neural tube defects, and low levels might suggest Down syndrome. (Patients who took the CVS test will take this one at about week 16 to test for spina bifida and other birth defects.)

Triple Screen test (at 18–20 weeks): The results from this blood draw are more precise than the AFP test (above). The triple screen measures AFP levels as well as levels of human chorionic gonadotropin (hCG) and estriol, a form of estrogen. The results are scrutinized for neural tube defects and

Down syndrome indicators. If results indicate either, an ultrasound or amniocentesis will follow for confirmation.

Quad Screen test (at 18–20 weeks): Most women opt for this group of tests since they are more precise than the triple screen. In addition to screening for inhibin-A levels, the quad screen provides results that, combined with the first trimester's nuchal translucency and PAPP-A blood test, generate the most accurate screening for Down syndrome and chromosomal abnormalities.

⊕ *DOC TALK: I remind patients that no tests for chromosomal abnormalities or birth defects are mandatory. Parents must make this decision for themselves. People hold many social, ethical, moral, and religious beliefs. I encourage them to think: "What will I do with the results?" Having a plan of action helps reduce anxiety.*

Body Building:
Signs Your Body Is Hard at Work

In addition to all the changes you may have begun to notice in the first trimester (breast changes; cramps; constipation and gassiness; faintness and palpitations; varicose veins and hemorrhoids; frequent urination), you may start to notice some additional minor and major discomforts. And remember, this is the *easy* trimester.

Increased hair and nail growth: Hormones are putting hair and nail production into high gear. Hair growth will be noticeable in places previously not hairy—or at least not *that* hairy. Waxing and tweezing may make you feel better, but in the meantime, enjoy having some of the best hair days of your life.

Bleeding gums: Increased blood volume can make your gums more sensitive to irritation and bleeding. Use a softer-bristled brush and brush more gently.

Heartburn: Hormones make digestion sluggish and relax the esophageal sphincter, allowing for a back-flow of stomach acids that can cause discomfort. Antacids offer quick relief and, as a bonus, provide calcium. Avoid spicy foods, which will exacerbate indigestion. Avoid supine positions immediately after eating. If you can't resist that late-night spicy Italian dinner with friends, just make sure it's a good one—you could be re-experiencing it for days.

Nosebleeds and congestion: Hormones cause swelling and increased blood flow to the blood vessels in your nose, which can lead to bleeding and stuffiness. Apply pressure or ice to nosebleeds.

Carpal tunnel syndrome: The nerve that runs through the wrist area can be squeezed by fluid retention. If there's enough compression on the nerve, tingling and numbness in the hand will occur. Wearing wrist splints will relieve some of the pressure and inflammation. As with many symptoms during pregnancy, this one will disappear soon after birth.

Skin changes: Hormones affect skin pigmentation by activating melanin cells. You may notice a darkening of the line between the pubic bone and bellybutton called *linea nigra*. It sounds sort of naughty, but it's actually just another weird, nonsexy condition. And talk about nonsexy: Some women also experience chloasma, known as the "cloak of pregnancy," in which brownish patches appear in a masklike pattern on the face. Moles, too, can darken and expand during pregnancy. Stay out of the sun to reduce melanin activity. Skin tags can crop up this trimester, too, as your skin cells feel the stimulating effects of your pregnancy hormones. Most of these changes will resolve after you give birth.

Stretch marks: These pinkish striations can crop up anywhere the skin is being stretched—bellies, breasts, butts, thighs. They are permanent but will eventually fade to a silvery hue.

"Pregnancy brain": Many women experience forgetfulness at this time. Your baby, body, and all the obligations surrounding prenatal care take up so much space in the brain that it can be a challenge to remember what day it is or where your sunglasses are or that you forgot your firstborn in the waiting room at your doctor's office.

Leukorrhea: This mucusy vaginal discharge is harmless and acts as a barrier to the cervix. If the discharge changes from whitish to a color, check with your doctor to make sure you have not developed an infection.

Leg cramps: A common complaint. Fluid retention and dehydration are thought to be the culprits, as well as the changes in a woman's center of gravity, which stresses the posterior compartment muscles in different ways. Basically, the body has to work harder to keep you upright. These compensations can lead to lower back pain, muscle spasms, upper back and shoulder pain, and hamstring and calf cramping. Stretch and massage the muscles to relieve cramping, especially before falling asleep and upon waking.

Dressing for Excess

When it comes to maternity clothes, expectant moms are often torn between vanity and practicality. You are already beginning to feel huge and uncomfortable, so some hip maternity clothes might brighten your spirits, right? But the price tags won't. Solutions? Try these:

[1] Splurge on a few key pieces that flatter your new figure and make you feel good.

[2] Raid the sale racks for marked-down larger-size clothing.

[3] Don't forget that you may have to buy as you go. You'll likely graduate from your early maternity clothes into even bigger maternity clothes as you start your final months, so plan your purchases accordingly.

[4] Remember that friends and relatives are keen to pass along maternity clothes. (You'll know this feeling as you outgrow those designer maternity jeans two weeks after buying them. You'll want someone to get your money's worth out of them.)

[5] Don't forget consignment shops for cheap, gently used items.

[6] A smart strategy is to invest in some basic, neutral pants, skirts, and tops and then create the illusion of a large wardrobe by rotating accessories (bags, eye-catching necklaces, bracelets or earrings, scarves, shoes). Here's another shopping rationalization (if you need one): Splurge on some high-end accessories since you'll be able to use them after you're back to your pre-baby self.

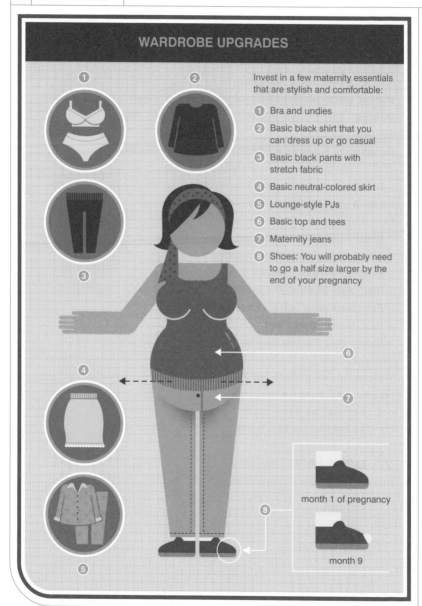

WARDROBE UPGRADES

Invest in a few maternity essentials that are stylish and comfortable:

1. Bra and undies
2. Basic black shirt that you can dress up or go casual
3. Basic black pants with stretch fabric
4. Basic neutral-colored skirt
5. Lounge-style PJs
6. Basic top and tees
7. Maternity jeans
8. Shoes: You will probably need to go a half size larger by the end of your pregnancy

month 1 of pregnancy

month 9

[7] As always, avoid horizontal stripes, large patterns, and poorly cut clothing, which only emphasize your girth. Black and dark colors really are slimming.

Consider the following wardrobe prescription:

■ Bra and undies for your new shape (either over the belly or bikini under-pants). A great-fitting bra—especially when you're pregnant—is essential for support and a put-together look.
■ Maternity jeans: Go for a slimming dark rinse. Avoid peg leg, matchstick, or "skinny" jeans; they will only emphasize your Humpty-Dumpty silhouette.
■ Basic top and tees (great for layering)
■ Basic black shirt that you can dress up or go casual
■ Basic black pants with stretch fabric
■ Basic neutral-colored skirt
■ Lounge-style PJs (put them on after work and don't take them off until morning)
■ Shoes: You will probably need to go a half size larger by the end of your pregnancy, so invest in a pair of sneakers and one pair of dress shoes. Slip-ons, of course, are much easier to deal with than lace-ups. You'll under-stand the first time you have to bend over your own firm girth to tie up laces.

⚠ **EXPERT TIP:** *You'll feel more like yourself if you shop the maternity lines of the brands you normally wear.*

Sleeping Skills—in Your Dreams

As your pregnant body grows, sleeping can feel like a new skill to be mastered. With heartburn, nasal congestion and snoring, leg cramps, increasing pressure on your diaphragm from your growing uterus, and your racing heart, you will likely join the ranks of the sleep deprived. (Consider it practice for all those nights to come when the little nipper will keep you up around the clock.)

Additionally, some expectant moms begin to feel aches in their hips and need to heave themselves from one side to the other throughout the night. Giant body pillows need to be resettled after each change. Diesel-powered pregnancy snoring revs up. And don't forget all those nighttime trips to the bathroom. At this point, partners will often give up and retreat to the sofa. Even family pets will think, "Screw it," and hop off the bed for quieter quarters.

Tips for Sleeping While Pregnant

[1] Sleep on your left side. Sleeping on your back is a no-no until delivery. If you lie flat, your growing uterus will compress the body's large blood vessels (the aorta and vena cava run through the chest and abdomen, along the spine) and thereby decrease the return of blood to your heart, which can in turn decrease blood flow to the baby. Rest assured, most women will start to feel the warning signs of a racing heart, shortness of breath, or dizziness long before any harm is done to the baby. Don't make yourself crazy about this side-sleeping thing. If you wake up on your back, just roll onto your side. Go left if you can.

[2] Employ pillow power. Some moms swear by an army of supportive pillows or one giant, full-length one to support the body where it's needed most.

While on your side, place the pillow between your knees. That will reduce the angle at which your leg descends from your hip, putting less stress on your hip and reducing residual aches. (Note: Your partner may be less fond of your giant pillow encroaching on his side of the bed.)

[3] Adjust your sleeping temperature. For optimum comfort, keep your bedroom at 72ºF (22ºC) or even cooler. Though a pregnant woman's baseline temperature does not differ significantly from that of a nonpregnant woman, her ability to dissipate heat does. Chalk it up to all those hormones and the baby.

[4] Exercise during the day. If you exert yourself during the day, your body should be ready for sleep at nighttime.

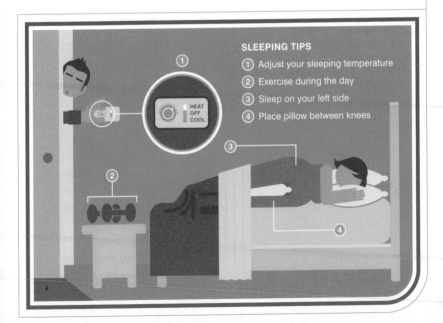

SLEEPING TIPS

① Adjust your sleeping temperature
② Exercise during the day
③ Sleep on your left side
④ Place pillow between knees

[5] Clean up sloppy sleep at night. If you are just lying in bed unable to sleep, you may want to get out of bed and read a book. Once you feel sleepy again, return to bed and try again. Do not take daytime naps—and certainly not late afternoon or early evening naps—until you're back in sleep synch.

⊕ *DOC TALK: I remind people that we used to live in caves, eat dirt, and get chased by wild animals, and the human race has persevered even without body pillows and sleeping on their left sides. So don't add "Am I sleeping the right way?" to your list of concerns. I don't really care which way you lean as long as you try to avoid sleeping flat.*

What to Do When You Get a Cold or Flu

Having a bad cold on top of your many pregnancy symptoms just does not seem fair. But take comfort that the antibodies your body produces to fight off a virus will cross the placenta and protect the baby as well. Baby will even keep these antibodies for a few weeks after delivery until it's time for him to make his own. A few things you *can* do:

▪ Get a flu shot (flu season can run October–May). Your baby will also carry flu immunity for the first several weeks after birth. Flu vaccination used to be recommended only after the first trimester, but now anytime in pregnancy is considered safe for mom and baby.

▪ Rest.

▪ Drink fluids.

▪ Use a humidifier to relieve congestion.

■ Call your doctor if you have a persistent, high fever or symptoms that do not resolve in three days.

■ Take appropriate medicine. Many over-the-counter meds are perfectly safe to use during pregnancy. (See sidebar, below.)

OK by the OB: Medications for Common Ailments

These readily available drugs are considered safe to take during your pregnancy, but since no medication can be completely safe for all women, be sure to check with your doctor first.

Allergy/cold: Diphenhydramine, Chlorpheniramine, Loratadine, Clemastine

Cough: Dextromethorphan

Congestion: Pseudoephedrine

Pain relief, headache, or fever: Acetominophen

Gas: Simethicone

Constipation: Fiber therapy, stool softeners (Docusate sodium), and laxatives

Hemorrhoids: 1% hydrocortisone cream

Insomnia: Diphenhydramine

⊕ DOC TALK: Many people find that they get sick more easily during pregnancy. That is entirely normal, since the body is under constant stress from less sleep, diet changes, and physical fatigue.

Traveling for Two

Some women must travel for work, and others will want one last romantic getaway before baby arrives. Travel is perfectly safe unless you are experiencing complications from a high-risk pregnancy—and even then, it's likely you can still travel somewhat.

Many doctors advise curtailing airplane trips after the 34th week so that if complications arise, you do not give birth away from home. There's nothing inherently dangerous about altitudes because the cabin is pressurized; air travel is no threat to breaking your water. (If you lose cabin pressure, you've got a lot more to worry about than your water bag.)

Airlines have different policies on how far along pregnant women can be and still board a plane. To avoid last-minute hassles, bring a note from your doctor approving your travel. Better to be overly prepared than waving forlornly at the jet you were supposed to be on as it taxis down the runway to your island getaway.

Travel Tips

[1] Choose a destination that has safe, clean accommodations, access to good medical care, and a well-equipped hospital.

[2] Save exotic adventures in foreign lands that require special shots and vaccines for later. Contracting dengue fever or cholera is probably not how you had envisioned your pregnancy.

[3] If traveling internationally, be wary of tap water and ice cubes. Drink purified bottled water instead.

[4] Always carry a complete and up-to-date medical history that includes the date your pregnancy began. Also make sure that you and your traveling companions know the accurate week of pregnancy you are in.

[5] Pack extra prenatal vitamins in case you get marooned at your destination or the airport.

[6] Pack extra snacks, too.

[7] If you're flying, confirm regulations for pregnant travelers before buying your ticket. Some airlines will not allow boarding after 36 weeks.

[8] When flying, make sure to stay hydrated. Air in planes is dry and can exacerbate pregnancy symptoms such as congestion. Try a little petroleum jelly in the nostrils.

[9] If you are traveling by plane, car, or train, make sure to take breaks from sitting in one position. It is vital to stave off deep vein thrombosis (DVT) by keeping blood circulating freely. (DVT leads to blood clots that may travel dangerously to the heart, lungs, or brain.) Avoid crossing your legs at the knees.

[10] As you did before your pregnancy, always wear a seat belt while in a car.

[11] If going by car, budget more time in your itinerary for pit stops (to stretch legs, eat, and use the rest room).

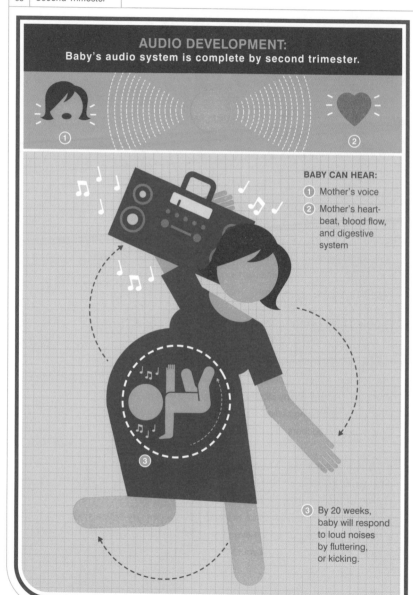

Baby, Can You Hear Me?

The answer is yes.

A baby's auditory system is complete by the second trimester. Studies have shown that the fetus can hear, and recognize, his or her mom's voice—though the sound waves will be dampened by travel through the abdominal and uterine walls and amniotic fluid. The growing baby is familiar with the background hum of all your internal system's workings, too. That's why there's a market for newborn sleep-aid products that replicate ambient amniotic sounds (whoosh, whoosh, whoosh). Babies are calmed by the familiar sounds of mom's digestive system, heartbeat, and blood flow. By 20 weeks baby will also respond to external stimuli (loud noises). You could notice a little flutter or kick if a loud siren goes by. Moms: Keep salty language to a minimum!

Block That Tummy Touch!

Who knows what goes through the minds of strangers, but they do seem to have an irresistible urge to touch pregnant women's protruding stomachs. Has there ever been a pregnant woman who wanted to be touched by a stranger? Unlikely. Many don't even want people they know—and love—touching their bulging bellies. Some suggestions to deter those oddly determined tummy touchers:

■ Try a little soft shoe. Turn slightly or take a step or two back from the offender. If they still come at you, they are more likely to get your arm instead of your tummy.

■ Keep talking. People tend not to make their move while in the middle of a conversation. So lock on the eye contact and do not stop blabbing.

■ Bend down suddenly to tie your shoe as soon as you recognize a tummy touch in the offing.

■ Fake an attack of violent coughing.

■ Wear a large coat to disguise your growing belly.

■ Deliver any of the following verbal rebukes:

• A polite, clipped "No thanks."

• "If you want to touch my tummy, I will touch yours first."

• "Do I know you?"

• "Oh no. My water is breaking." (People don't want amniotic fluid on their shoes and will back off immediately.)

• Just holler, "Hands off!"

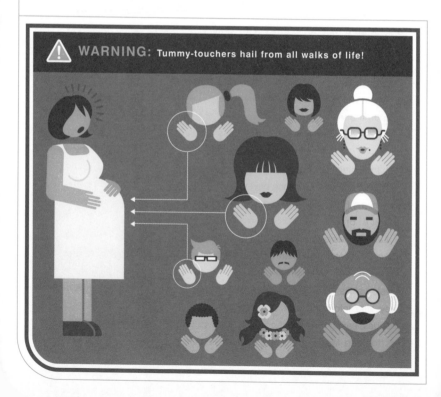

Get Some Class: Birthing, Baby Care, and Breast-Feeding

Many first-time pregnant women have no idea what they're in for. Fortunately, there's help for them, and even for second-time-around moms who need refreshers. Birthing, baby-care, and breast-feeding classes can demystify the mysterious new reality that is about to unfold.

Birthing class: Typically these are taught by registered nurses with extensive experience in labor and delivery. Some are ongoing, whereas others are a one-day crash course. At hospital-sponsored classes, you and your birthing coach usually receive a tour of the birthing facilities and learn about normal stages of labor, Cesarean sections, pain medications, labor-relaxation techniques, and what to pack for your hospital or birthing center stay. Take this opportunity to ask questions of a nurse who has been in the trenches.

Natural childbirth classes: The two best-known natural childbirth methods (meaning no drugs and no medical interventions, if possible) are *Lamaze*, named after French physician Fernand Lamaze, and *Bradley*, also known as Husband-Coached Childbirth, named after American doctor Robert A. Bradley.

Lamaze has been around the longest and has the greatest name recognition. The natural childbirth method champions a woman's ability to give birth using inner wisdom to guide her through the rigors of labor. Classes develop skills to decrease pain and discomfort and speed labor and birth. They also inform you about labor support, exercise, breathing, position changes, eating and drinking, aromatherapy, hydrotherapy, and other methods to keep Mom relaxed and labor progressing. Families are educated about appropriate medical interventions so that laboring women can work as informed decision makers with their health care providers.

The Bradley method strongly discourages medication, instead emphasizing a woman's powerful ability to give birth naturally when strengthened by her partner's loving support. Moms cite its muscle-relaxation techniques as being highly effective in the heat of labor. Bradley classes also discuss nutrition and other aspects of pregnancy and childbirth. Classes meet for 12 two-hour sessions.

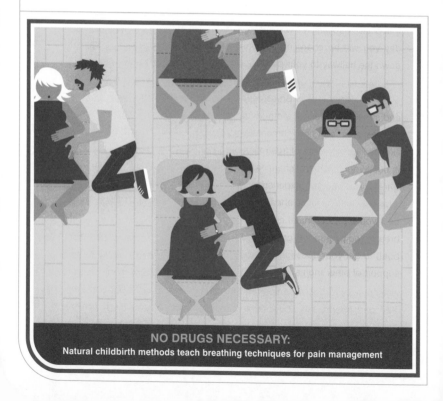

NO DRUGS NECESSARY:
Natural childbirth methods teach breathing techniques for pain management

All natural childbirth prep classes emphasize that birth is a normal, natural, and healthy process and that it can be experienced free of routine medical intervention. Natural childbirth can profoundly affect and empower women and their families. Women who deliver their babies without medication frequently find the experience exhilarating.

Baby-care class: This type of class is suited for the parent who, until now, has had little opportunity to interact with babies—and thus may have a good deal of trepidation about the new skill set required once she's home with baby. On the syllabus are diapering, bathing, and other basics. If diapering that plastic baby leaves you in a fretful sweat, take comfort knowing that one day you will be changing the baby, talking on the phone, and shouting down the hallway to your partner about dinner plans all at the same time.

Breast-feeding class: Breast-feeding is a beautiful, but often perplexing and stressful, aspect of motherhood. Though natural and considered to be the best source of nourishment for your child, it is not easy at first. You will likely spill many tears of frustration until you and your baby get the hang of it; but if you persevere, chances are you'll feel it was worth it, having gained a treasured bonding experience. If you plan to breast-feed, get as much information as possible ahead of time. Your caregiver should be able to connect you with a prenatal class. Once you have delivered your child, join a breast-feeding support group (also a great way to meet moms in the same boat) to get your questions answered. First-timers will have many, and the support of other moms and breast-feeding veterans is invaluable.

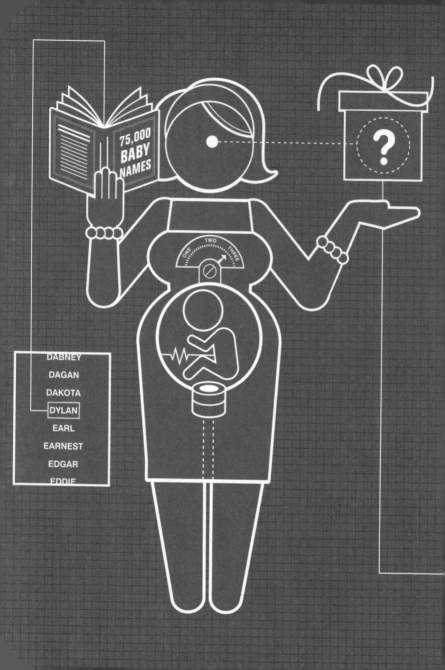

Chapter 4

Third Trimester

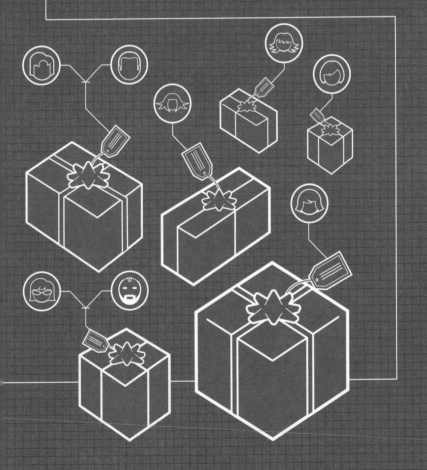

By the third trimester, many a gal is awash in minor physical discomforts. You're huge, you ache, you pee, you pee some more, you snore, and so on. But you have also learned to adapt. You may complain (a lot at times), but really you're taking it in stride. And you're starting to get really, really excited and filled with heart-racing anticipation of soon holding your baby and looking into his eyes. "So that's who you are!"

It's something to make your knees quake in wonder and awe—especially since your ligaments are already so loose from all those hormones. This last trimester is all about building suspense for the big day that's fast approaching.

When you do meet your child, be prepared for some waterworks. With hormones recalibrating after delivery, it's inevitable—especially when you tenderly cradle your baby inches from your own face, search every little curve, dimple, and pore of his angelic visage, and feel the touch of his soft skin and inhale his milky smell. This bond is a fierce and astonishing one. We mothers are lucky to experience it. (You'll want to keep that in mind at the 4 A.M. feeding, when exhaustion penetrates every cell and fiber of your being.)

So get ready because he, she, or they are almost here.

Synopsis of Baby's Growth, Weeks 27–40+

Your baby's systems are all in place and are now simply maturing in preparation for birth. She is developing layers of fat that will help her regulate her temperature after birth. Your baby is considered full term by week 37 and postterm if she is still in utero beyond week 42. Some form of testing is advised beyond week 41 to ensure that the placenta is still functioning adequately and providing the baby with enough oxygen and nutrients. Most doctors recommend induction after 42 weeks because the placenta is likely running out of gas, and for the baby's health, you don't want that to happen suddenly.

Seeing Your Caregiver in the Third Trimester; or, Who's Your New Best Friend?

In your third trimester, your prenatal visits will increase to every two to three weeks starting at the 32-week point. Many then become weekly around week 34 or 35. These visits are useful for the doctor since he or she can distinguish between your normal third trimester discomforts and true complications, such as gestational diabetes and hypertension.

In addition to giving you any needed pep talks, sound advice, wise anecdotes, or simple contradictions to ridiculous urban legends or myths about childbirth, the doctor will check:

- Weight
- Blood pressure
- Urine
- Edema (fluid retention) on ankles and hands
- Baby's heartbeat
- Location of the fundus (top of the uterus) to monitor fetal growth

Baby's Growth, Weeks 27–40+

WEEK		
27 through **33**	✓ Develops sense of smell	✓ Puts on baby fat
	✓ Weighs about 3 pounds (1.5 kg)	✓ More than 15 inches (38 cm) long
	✓ Can open and close eyes	✓ Can follow a light with eyes
34 through **36**	✓ Weighs about 5 pounds (2.25 kg)	✓ Increase in fat rounds out body
	✓ Lungs are well developed	✓ Receives antibodies from the mother to protect from illness
37	➡ CONSIDERED FULL TERM	
38 through **39**	✓ More than 19 inches (48 cm) long*	
	✓ Weighs about 7 pounds (3 kg)*	
	*NOTE: Babies' sizes and weights can vary greatly at this stage.	
40	➡ READY FOR BIRTH	

Considered postterm if still in utero beyond week 42. Testing is advised beyond week 41 to ensure the placenta is functioning correctly.

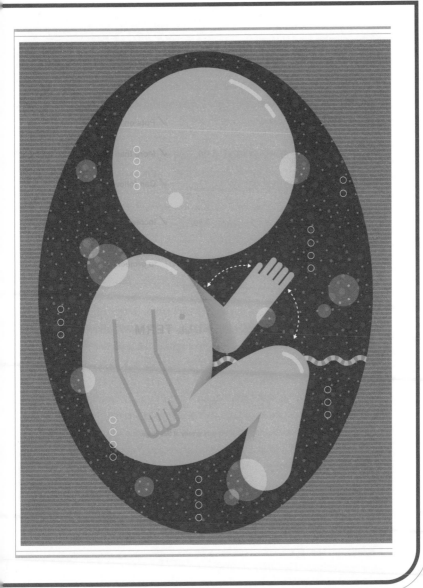

Additional Examination Topics

For the next few weeks, your doctor will also add a few more checks, just to keep things interesting. These new exams herald the beginning of the homestretch!

CERVICAL EXAM. From week 35 on, some doctors will check the state of the expectant mom's cervix to determine whether it is readying for delivery. The cervix begins the pregnancy as a firm, solid cylinder, but as the third trimester progresses and babies get larger and contractions begin, the cylinder starts to change. The doctor will be looking for:

■ the widening of the narrow canal that runs through the cervix.
■ thinning of the cervix, which usually starts at about four centimeters long and eventually becomes paper-thin during active labor.
■ changes in the "station" of the baby, which refers to the baby's position in the pelvis. Generally, babies will start high in the pelvis, which is termed a "minus station," but as contractions increase in intensity and frequency, babies move down to a "plus station." (When a baby is at "+3 station," she is at the opening of the vagina.)

Be aware, however, that even though the doctor may report no dilation or softening of the cervix, the situation may change at any time over the next few weeks. An added benefit of the exam is that it helps you put into context the cramps and contractions and pressure you feel with your doctor's assessment of the state of the cervix.

FETAL MOVEMENT. Your doctor will also ask you how much movement your baby is generating. Fetal movement is a good predictor of well-being because a baby who has plenty of oxygen and nutrients will be active. Many practitioners will ask you to keep track of movement with a "kick count."

The Kicks That Count

When your doctor asks you to keep track of your baby's movements, you will be monitoring for ten kicks an hour, two times a day.

[1] Since babies in utero have sleep cycles just like newborns, count after meals or before your bedtime. These are the times when your baby is most likely awake.

[2] Lie down and get comfy. Place your hands directly on your abdomen.

[3] Start counting. You can quit after you feel ten movements, even if you're done in five minutes. Movements tend to get more subtle as pregnancy progresses and the baby moves lower into the pelvis. Babies are less likely to do flips, but you can still feel shifting or twisting.

[4] If the kick count falls below ten kicks an hour or you do not feel any movement, contact your doctor.

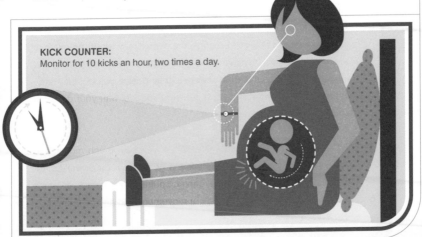

KICK COUNTER:
Monitor for 10 kicks an hour, two times a day.

Common Late-Term Complications

Complications can develop for some women as their bodies try to manage the increasing demands of a progressing pregnancy.

■ Hypertension and preeclampsia. This condition affects the kidneys and constricts blood flow to the fetus; it typically develops sometime after the 20th week. Signs of hypertension include edema, sudden weight gain, and protein in the urine. Common treatment includes rest, preferably on one side, to lower blood pressure.

■ Preterm labor. Labor is considered preterm if it occurs before the 37th week. Every day that a baby can continue to mature in the womb is critical, so your doctor will work to stop labor if it begins too soon. The first measure is bed rest. Medicines called tocolytics can be given to relax muscles and slow or prevent labor. If your baby is coming before 34 weeks of gestation despite all measures to stop him, doctors will administer a steroid to speed the maturation of the baby's lungs.

■ Gestational diabetes. Hormones can render insulin ineffective and produce high glucose levels in the blood. Women can use exercise and diet to control this condition, which should clear up after birth. If the condition cannot be treated with behavior modification, the mom may have to take insulin. The hazards of untreated gestational diabetes are babies who are too big for a smooth delivery and babies who will be encumbered with their own resulting health problems.

Third-Trimester Tests

■ Group B streptococcus (GBS) test (around 35 or 36 weeks). Your practitioner should test you for group B strep. Doctors recommend this test because newborn pediatricians have found that an overwhelming percentage of newborn infections (pneumonia, meningitis, sepsis) were caused by GBS. Approximately 25 percent of women have this bacterium in their vagina or rectum. (These are normally occurring bacteria and are not sexually transmitted.) If the bacterium is detected, you may be treated with a round of antibiotics; but if the bacteria have colonized, a simple course of medication won't do the trick. You will need to take antibiotics during delivery (through an IV line) to prevent the spread of the bacteria to your baby as she passes through the birth canal. Hey, the upside of a C-section is no worries about GBS!

⊕ DOC TALK: *Even if moms were not treated for Group B strep at all, the chances of its affecting the baby are still small. Sometimes we jump through a lot of hoops to prevent a small chance of problems.*

■ Non Stress Test, or the NST. This test is given for varied reasons including underlying maternal health problems, such as diabetes, hypertension, asthma, or chronic diseases like lupus, and such fetal conditions as compromised growth, amniotic fluid issues, or questions about movement.

Basically, you will monitor the baby's heart rate in conjunction with uterine activity to see that it is "reactive." But the non stress test might as well be labeled a "real stress test" for all the potential worry it can cause pregnant moms whose fetuses blissfully sleep through the whole exam. Just like babies outside the womb, babies in utero go through sleep cycles, and when babies are sleeping, they don't show the same reactivity on the monitoring as when they are awake. Sometimes the evaluator will even use an acoustic stimulator (like an alarm clock) to wake the baby. Don't worry: A monitoring session that is nonreactive is common and does not mean that your baby is in trouble, only that further testing is needed. Here's what to expect:

[**1**] You will lie in a comfy chair with a lead attached around your middle and a monitor resting on your uterus.

[**2**] The lead is connected to the fetal-heart–monitoring device, which will measure the baby's heartbeats and generate a paper readout for the practitioner to evaluate.

[**3**] For about 20 minutes, you'll simply remain in the chair, listening to the comforting, hypnotic sounds of your baby's heartbeat. Be sure to bring some reading material to pass the time—distractions are sometimes welcome so that you don't find yourself raising your own heart rate while craning to see what the spikes on the readout reveal.

[**4**] From time to time, the technician monitoring the test may use the acoustic stimulator near your belly to set off a little alarm-clock-like noise to wake baby if she appears to be sleeping.

[**5**] Once the technician has enough data, you will be able to sit up and remove the monitoring equipment.

[**6**] The technician or doctor will be looking for two accelerations in the fetal heart rate within a 20-minute period, with each acceleration 15 beats above the baby's baseline rate and lasting for 15 seconds. The changes in the heart rate indicate that the baby's central nervous system is intact and regulating and modulating her organ systems.

[**7**] If the results are "reactive"—that is, if baby's heart rate has shown the expected accelerations—you're good to go. But even if your doctor determines that the results are "nonreactive," that does not mean anything is

amiss. It may simply mean baby is still sleeping, in which case a longer monitoring session may be required or a more detailed exam, called "the biophysical profile" (an ultrasound session during which the physician examines baby's muscle movements, breathing, and amniotic fluid levels) will be administered as a follow-up.

Woman at Work: Construction Nearing Completion

By this point, you will no longer even recall how your body felt before pregnancy. The curious result will be a minimizing of some of your discomforts because they now seem entirely normal. That said, get ready: Many of your symptoms will increase in severity. Heartburn, fatigue, constipation, stretch marks, hemorrhoids, and snoring will only intensify. Keep in mind that your growing uterus is now fighting it out with your other organs for space. Its considerable size is compressing your colon, bladder, lungs, stomach, veins, and nerves—all of which will make sustained sleep more difficult.

Some women continue their normal routines up to the day of labor, but others find their usual activities significantly limited. Don't worry if you need lots of rest periods throughout the day. There are no pregnancy prizes for how grueling we can make our work schedule before delivery. Much will depend on the position your baby has chosen to nestle in.

⊕ *DOC TALK: At this stage, moms-to-be may feel great one day and miserable the next. One day they might have sciatic nerve pain shooting down the back of the legs and the next day suffer kicks in the ribs. It can be frustrating, especially for younger moms who are not used to physical limita-*

tions. But it is one of the first revelations of what it means to be a parent: You're now experiencing something completely out of your control, and the actions of that little body are affecting your life. It's a tough lesson!

Here are some of the other less-than-enjoyable symptoms you might experience:

- Fluid retention (edema), especially in the feet and hands
- Aches due to ligament stretching
- Loss of balance due to shifting center of gravity
- Abdominal muscle separation (rectus diathesis): As your uterus grows, your abdominal muscles begin to separate along the midline to make space for the baby. You don't really feel it, but when you sit up you may notice a bulge in your midsection that wasn't there before. (Your muscles will be back to their old shape pretty much six months after you deliver.)
- General discomfort: Serious grumpiness and moodiness pervade daily life, and it's little wonder: Your sleep quality is gone, eating even small meals kicks up heartburn, your breathing is shallow, your backaches increase, your bladder control diminishes, your vaginal pressure and discharge increase, and your ankles and feet swell.

Some Issues to Occupy Your Mind While Your Body Works Overtime

There are some issues you will want to research and put some thought into during these last weeks before baby arrives. Some need to be hashed out in preparation for delivery; others are longer term, such as selecting daycare, nannies, pediatricians, and so forth.

Name That Baby

There are cultural, regional, familial, and religious reasons that people choose a particular name for their child. There are personal, irrational, and highly subjective reasons that people choose a particular name for their child. Whatever imperative is at work, one mandate should be clear: Never, ever tell anyone the name you are considering for your child.

If you do, many curious well-wishers will quickly begin offering opinions on the name. It's rare that these comments will persuade you to change your mind. It's simpler to say, "We're keeping the name to ourselves until the baby arrives." Or just as truthfully, "We're not sure yet."

Here are some considerations for making your selection:

■ Nicknames. If you name your child William, are you comfortable with Bill or Willie? It may be out of your control when your son decides to adopt (or is given) a nickname. Same with Elizabeth: Be prepared to end up with Betty, Betsy, Liz, or Bette.

■ Initials. Pay attention to what the child's initials will be. Peter Ethan Evans (P.E.E.) may wish his parents had opted for Stanley.

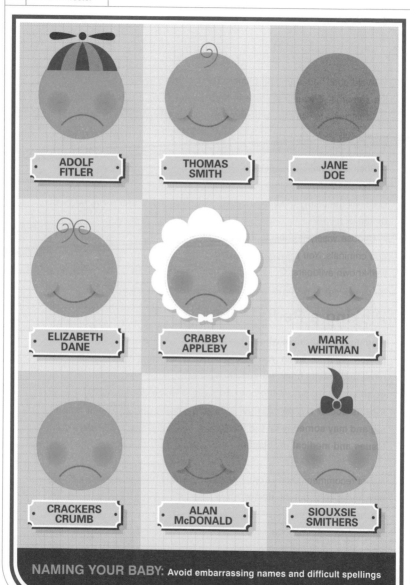

NAMING YOUR BABY: Avoid embarrassing names and difficult spellings

■ Avoid contrived-sounding names. Think of how the first name goes with the surname. If your last name is Kane, avoid Candace. Remember, your child will have to use this name through all stages of life, not just when she's a cute roly-poly baby. If your last name is Payne, avoid Helmut or Hart. Think: Will I still be laughing after my epidural has worn off?

■ Spell it normally. It's unkind to burden a child with a difficult or unusual spelling of a simple name. Stick with the basics and rest easy that your child will get plenty of chances in life to show how unique and creative he or she is.

■ Choose wisely if considering a name associated with tyrants, despots, and criminals. You may want to avoid giving your child a name shared by well-known evildoers. Or just people you and your partner don't like.

Picking a Pediatrician

Finding a pediatrician whom you like and trust is essential to your happiness. Just as when you selected an obstetrician or midwife, you'll need to do some homework. Your life will be exponentially easier if you do this legwork before the baby arrives. Take the assignment seriously, for this doctor will be your guide through the virgin territory of parenting and may someday be the trusted expert your child talks to about life issues and medical problems.

■ Get recommendations from your caregiver and friends. Ask what specifically they like about the doctor.

■ Check references.

■ Set up an informational session. This first contact can provide information about how you'll reach office staff when you really need them.

■ Get there early and pay attention to the waiting room. Do parents seem content or fed up? Is it run efficiently? Are the nurses or front-office staff happy to be there or complaining loudly? Is it clean? Are the children separated for sick and well visits? Strike up a conversation with other waiting parents and ask their opinions.

■ Interview the doctor. Possible questions include:

Will my child see you or a nurse practitioner?

- How fast can my child get an appointment when sick?
- How long do you take to return a call?
- Does the practice have a 24-hour help line?
- Does the doctor have weekend hours?
- At which hospital do you have privileges?
- What's your opinion on the dangers of the MMR vaccine and the question of its links to autism? (Regardless of your own feelings on vaccination, this hot-button issue should get your doctor talking, revealing her position on topics at the forefront of pediatric health.)
- What's your feeling on late-bloomers (babies who hit their milestones later than usual) and when parents should be concerned? (This question should give you a sense of how proactive the doctor is about early interventions and therapies for children who fall off the continuum of normal behavioral development.)

Once you have made your decision, inform your obstetrician or midwife of the doctor's name so that the pediatrician will be contacted after your baby is born.

⊕ DOC TALK: *Your choice is not set in stone. You are free to change pediatricians at any time. Doctors realize that parents may prefer someone who is a better "fit." Shop around till you're satisfied.*

Is It Time for a Personal Staff?

Once you have selected a pediatrician, ask yourself if you need or would like other experts in your life. Hard to believe you have arrived at this point, but you may soon find your simple life overrun with paid and essential professionals. Are you interested in natural childbirth? Then consider hiring a birth doula, a woman experienced in childbirth who can provide advice and support before and during childbirth. Desperate for some help when you bring home the baby? Consider a baby nurse or postdelivery doula. Going back to work in three months? Think nanny or daycare. While you're at it, you may welcome a biweekly cleaning service. As with your searches for an obstetrician or midwife and pediatrician, each search requires a multipronged approach: Get recommendations, conduct interviews, check references.

Do You Doula?

■ If you are looking for a doula, begin well in advance of your due date since many doulas are quickly booked up.

■ Contact all references. Ask what kind of support the doula provided. How did she work with the nursing staff and doctor? Did she include the partner in the labor and birth? Was she sensitive to the mom's changing moods? Did she know how to motivate the mom? What pain control measures did she use, and did she have specific methods for avoiding an episiotomy?

■ After you have done your research over the phone, set up in-person interviews. It is important that the two of you "click." When you're in the throes of labor, you will want a doula who intuitively understands you. Remember to ask the doula about her education and training as well as how many other clients she has around the time of your due date and what her contingency plans are in case she ends up with another mom delivering when you go into labor.

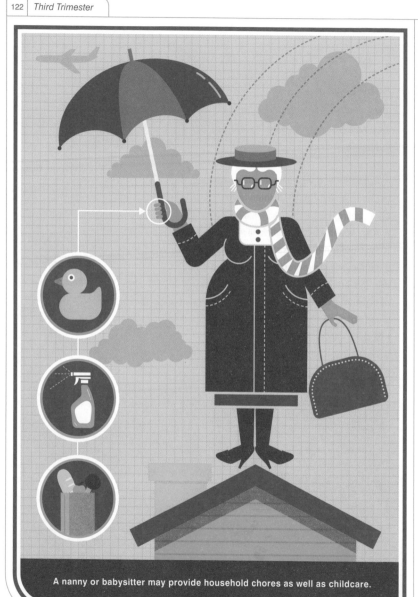

A nanny or babysitter may provide household chores as well as childcare.

Baby Daycare

If you have hired a pediatrician at this stage, you may want to ask him or her for daycare recommendations. You can also ask friends and neighbors for referrals and then:

- Research and visit all potential sites.
- Set up an informational interview and a tour. (An impromptu visit can also be revealing.)
- Ask for names of parents willing to speak about the facility.
- Find out the daycare's rules and schedules, the child-teacher ratio, what the educational program will be for your child, who has access to the building, the educational background of its staffers, whether they have done background checks on all employees, what their sick-child policy is, the length of time the child must stay home until recovered, and how they resolve conflict among children.
- Look to see that the facility is clean and safe and that the environment is welcoming, fun, and organized.

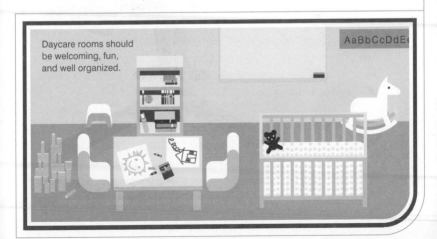

Daycare rooms should be welcoming, fun, and well organized.

AaBbCcDdE

Warning! Pre-Labor Ahead

In the pre-labor warmup, your body can experience changes indicating that birth is approaching. Women can feel these signs, which occur in the weeks leading up to delivery, with varying degrees of severity, or they may not feel them at all.

Braxton-Hicks contractions: These uterine muscular contractions begin early in pregnancy, though they are not particularly noticeable until you are well along. You will notice a tightening, or tensed-muscle feeling, of your entire uterus. The contractions are brief and painless. Sometimes they occur in a cluster, but unlike real labor, they will stop. Closer to delivery, Braxton-Hicks contractions can help ripen the cervix (see "Doc Talk" below).

DOC TALK: It is difficult for a woman to differentiate between Braxton-Hicks and labor contractions. In the third trimester, false labor pains are more intense and frequent with the mom's increased activity and dehydration. If you feel contractions, find a cool place and put up your feet, drink fluids, and rest. If the contractions space out and lessen in intensity, then it is usually false labor. If they become more frequent and intense, especially if they occur every five minutes, call your doctor. I remind patients that no one ever delivered a baby and described the sensation as "crampy." The intensity of what it takes to make the baby come through the birth canal is usually described as so strong they "can't walk or talk."

Dilation and effacement: Think of your cervix as though it were a big, plump bagel. This bagel, all closed up tight, will begin to thin and spread in preparation for delivery. This dilation (opening) and effacement (flattening) can happen over weeks, in a day, or within hours. There is no standard timeframe, and no way is more auspicious than another. As your due date approaches, you will be given numbers by your practitioner, such as "2 centimeters dilated, 1 centimeter effaced."

"Lightening": This phenomenon happens when the baby drops down into the pelvic cradle and is "engaged" (meaning the baby is no longer floating around). Braxton-Hicks contractions often move the baby down into the pelvis. Think of it as though the baby were getting into the blast-off position. When this shift happens varies greatly, and some women do not experience it until actual labor. For many women, lightening is a good news/bad news scenario. Breathing and eating are easier now that the baby has shifted south, but pressure on the bladder and pelvic ligaments increase bathroom trips and, for some, create a sensation that the baby will drop out because he or she is riding so low. Your practitioner will know by an internal exam how far the baby is into your pelvis, or his or her "station."

Nesting: Not Just for the Birds

Pregnant women often experience a strong desire to prepare a "nest" before the onset of labor, and for some this behavior begins even earlier. The surge of "nesting" energy, which contrasts strongly with the more typical weary state of the final trimester, compels moms-to-be to transform their living environments into cozy incubators of neatness and organization. Another condition of "nesting" is the urgency and focus with which you must complete

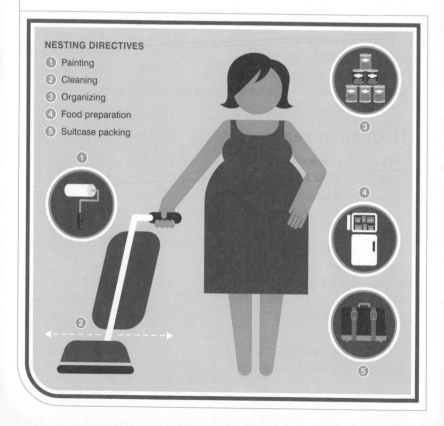

NESTING DIRECTIVES
1. Painting
2. Cleaning
3. Organizing
4. Food preparation
5. Suitcase packing

tasks as well as your demands that family members comply immediately with your wishes. Nesting is commonly directed toward such activities as:

- painting, cleaning, and arranging the nursery
- eliminating unnecessary clutter
- organizing like items (food in pantry, books, tools in garage, photos)
- overall home cleanliness or finishing major home projects
- procuring and arranging baby clothing
- baking and cooking food for freezer storage
- packing suitcase for hospital

Important caveat: Some pregnant women never experience "nesting," or if they do they are too slothful to act upon it with any noticeable vigor.

Nothing to Fear but Labor Itself

Many women experience anxiety about labor. As your due date approaches, so do worries about everything going smoothly, particularly the well-being of you and your baby.

Here are some techniques to control your anxiety.

[1] Educate yourself. Ask your doctor, nurse, or experienced moms to walk you through the whole process, with all the details. Labor is a natural process and one that produces your baby. Pain is merely a byproduct. Fear begets fear, so stop that cycle and learn about what your body is doing to achieve your baby's delivery.

[2] Assemble a good labor team. By taking charge and getting organized, you will be able to relax and direct your energy to the right tasks. Pick

labor coaches you trust (typically selected from your inner circle of confidants, including your partner, sisters, mom, or close friends). They will be in the delivery room to offer support, distraction, or anything you need. Check with your practitioner to see if there are limits on how many people can be with you in the delivery room.

[3] Write a birth plan. The exercise of writing down the desired conditions for the birth of your child may empower you. This is the document that one of your labor coaches will share with the medical staff on duty when you arrive at the hospital or birthing center. It may specify your feeling about pain medicine or birth positions. You may very well end up overturning every wish on your list, but at least you'll have thought things over in advance.

➕ *DOC TALK: You can make all the birth plans in the world, but I like to remind patients that labor is a dynamic process that can go on for days. Many variables can change in an instant, the biggest one being how the baby tolerates labor. So stay flexible. If things are progressing appropriately, then minimal, if any, interventions are needed. However, even in the healthiest and most prepared and educated patients, sometimes things occur that might necessitate interventions and even a C-section. I try to focus patients on one thought: The only thing that matters is that Mom and baby are healthy. The rest is secondary.*

[4] Visualize the process. Run through it from start to finish, from leaving your home to returning with a gorgeous, healthy baby. Make a movie in your mind of your successful, calm, and relaxed birth process. Play it over in your head whenever worries crop up. Even throw in an event that forces you to deviate from your birth plan and then imagine yourself rolling with the change, ending up with a happy baby in your arms.

[5] Investigate alternative therapies. Acupuncture has been used to relieve everything from morning sickness to labor pain. Acupuncture needles are placed at strategic points on the body and are thought to release endorphins that remedy the area of concern. Self-hypnosis can also be a valuable skill for calming an expectant mother. Hypnosis targets fears when the body is in an extremely receptive state. Used with autosuggestion (repeating a phrase till you believe it, such as, "I will have a calm, healthy birth"), hypnosis may help you face your anxieties with more confidence. You will need to practice ahead of time if you wish to use self-hypnosis successfully.

JUST FOR DADS: Men are going through almost all the same anxieties and fears that Mom is, minus the physical discomforts. Getting through labor will likely be the hardest thing you'll witness your partner experience. Be prepared by reading books and don't be afraid to watch several episodes of those birthing shows instead of SportsCenter.

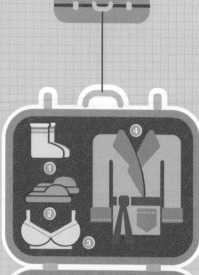

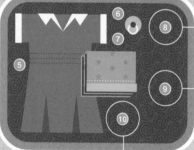

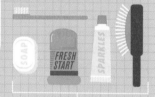

SUPPLIES LIST

1. Socks
2. Slippers
3. Nursing bra
4. Robe
5. Going-home outfit
6. Pacifiers (just in case)
7. Swaddling blanket
8. Toiletries
9. Reading material
10. List of phone numbers to call to share the happy news

SOAP

FRESH START

SPARKLES

baby
owner's manual

Mom's cell
555-176-9292
Uncle Dale's cell
555-454-8881
Mr. Bentley
555-686-9000
Cousin Collin
555-432-1776

PACKING FOR D-DAY!

Start Your Engines: A Labor Prep Checklist

This is the trimester when you need to be ready to roll, and roll quickly. Take the time to prepare so that by the last month you have no worries.

☑ Pack your bag and have it ready at the door by week 37. Include socks and slippers, robe, nursing bras, a going-home outfit for you (your maternity clothes may still be required) and for baby, a swaddling blanket, pacifiers (just in case), toiletries, reading material, and a list of phone numbers to call to share the happy news.

Most hospitals provide gowns, which will be your uniform while there, and "underwear," a disposable, fishnetlike undergarment to which you will affix gigantic sanitary pads to absorb postpartum locchia (bleeding, and lots of it). So save room in your suitcase for baby's first teddy bear and leave your pretty nightgowns and extra undies at home.

☑ Consider a separate tote bag for gear you may want to bring along, including music, pillows, therapy balls, brushes, massage lotions and tools, aromatherapy items, photographs of beloved pets or other images that will trigger a sense of calm, snacks for those who are allowed to eat, change for vending machines, and camera or recording equipment.

☑ Buy and install a rear-facing car seat suitable for a newborn.

☑ Pick labor coaches. Confirm how many support team members are allowed in the delivery room. If you have more than allowed, consider rotating them in and out of the room.

☑ Figure out contact strategies for family and friends. Do you want your entire family in the hospital waiting room? Do you want them there only after the baby has arrived? Do you want some but not all? Some may want to visit when you are rested and settled. Be clear about who will be in the delivery room and who will have to wait outside. This is your time to call the shots, and if someone gets offended just blame it on "pregnancy hormones."

☑ Establish a phone tree. Designate a sibling to call extended family or your best friend to call your circle of friends. If you intend to make the calls, make sure you take a list of phone numbers to the hospital. Have your closest colleague spread the word at work or have your partner send out an e-mail blast.

☑ Pack your birth plan. (See p. 128.) This is a document the staff at your hospital or birthing center will read to understand your wishes for the birthing process. It will help the trained professionals around you understand how best to meet your goals and how to encourage you.

The Baby Shower

Baby showers are typically hosted by a close friend or relative of the expectant mom in the final trimester, when she is far along and the pregnancy safely established. The purpose is to celebrate the expectant mom, remind her that she has a circle of friends who will support her in her upcoming role, and load her up with some adorable baby gear. The type of party can range from an elegant tea party to a rollicking (virgin) margarita fest, and anything in between. The following instructions are meant for your baby shower host. Copy the list below and review it with the trusted friend or relative organizing the event.

■ Schedule the party about a month or two from due date so that the guest of honor still has energy.

■ Plan on the festivities being fairly brief since most third-trimester moms may not have the stamina they used to. Two hours is a good target.

■ Whoever sends out the invitations may want to include baby registry information. Crass? Perhaps. Most guests will appreciate the information anyway.

THROWING A PROPER BABY SHOWER

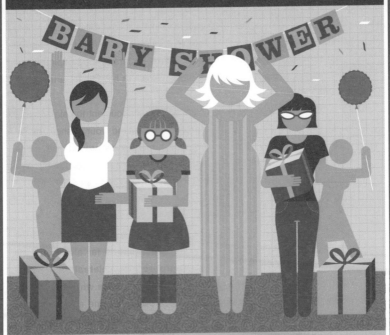

TIPS FOR THROWING A SHOWER

1. Schedule the party about a month before the due date
2. Include baby registry information with invite
3. Keep the food with shower's theme
4. Devise games and reward the winners with a nice prize
5. Keep the festivities fairly brief
6. Blank journal where guests can write will become a prized keepsake

■ Showers used to be reserved for the women, but now spouses and male friends regularly show up. Bear in mind, however, that a lot of men would rather spend their two hours elsewhere rather than listening to a bunch of women squealing over tiny baby clothes. They may thank you for making it a testosterone-free event.

■ If your guest of honor feels uncomfortable with the notion of inviting a bunch of friends over to give her stuff, turn the tables. Devise a guessing game or contest and reward the winners with spa treatments or some other treat. Also, make sure guests walk away with a nice bag of party favors: pink or blue candies, a small plant, baked goods, or manicure certificates.

■ Keep the food with your theme, but remember to include some bland items for your guest of honor, who may be unable to tolerate anything with a strong taste. Keep a bottle of antacids on hand.

■ Silly games tend to define these events, but consider displaying a blank journal where guests can write down "best" advice, memories, or other warm wishes. It will definitely become a prized keepsake.

■ Play games as an icebreaker before the meal is served.

■ Round out the event with the gift-opening festivities. Help the mom-to-be by designating someone to keep a list of gifts and their givers to make thank-you notes easy.

Getting Through Your Baby Shower

Although you may be feeling like a shower is the last thing you want, you'll certainly look back with fond memories on the gathering—and likely get some good stuff, too! Some helpful tips for the guest of honor:

[1] Rest up beforehand. Take a nap or sleep late that morning. Though you will certainly be excused from standing a lot, you may miss out on some

of the good gossip and conversation if you restrict yourself to the corner lounge chair.

[2] Wear sensible shoes: By now you're heavily pregnant. It would be a shame to suffer shoe pain by trying to squeeze into your designer heels one last time.

[3] Don't panic if you forget good friends' names. Pregnancy brain is likely to attack when you are making multiple introductions. Just laugh it off.

[4] Do eat. If the food is tasty, dig in. You've never had a better excuse to chow down at a party. It's also important to keep your blood-sugar levels steady.

[5] Use your compromised bladder as an excuse to get out of anything you don't feel like doing. If a friend tries to rope you into one of the gross melted-chocolate-candy-bar-in-the-diaper games, plead a full bladder and beat it to the bathroom.

[6] Thank everyone for coming. Though you may be pooped by the end of the party, thank each person warmly. You may not see them for a while.

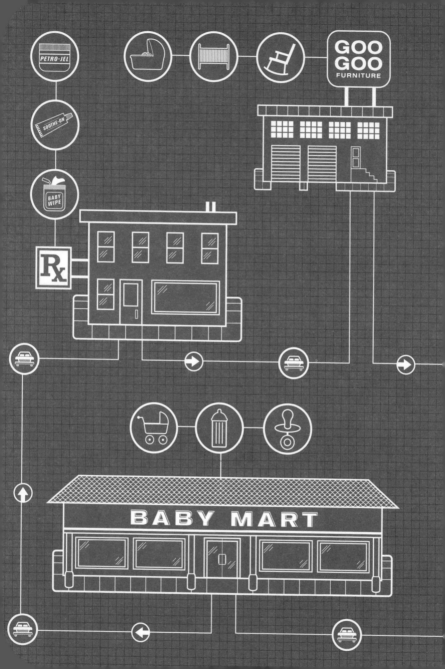

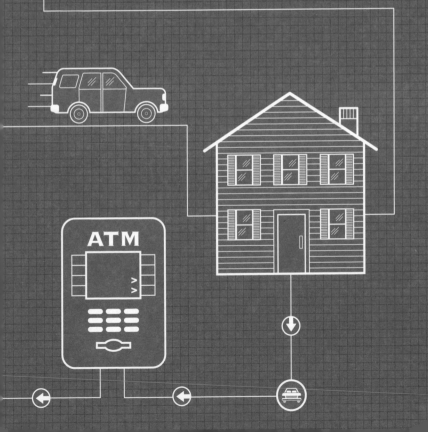

Chapter 5

Layette
and Nursery

ATM

You may think that you need to have every single thing set up in the nursery before the baby arrives, but here's the reality: You don't. In fact, once your baby has arrived, you may be surprised to find that he needs a lot of a certain thing (bibs, if he spits up a lot) and not so much of another (all those cute tiny socks are fairly useless if he's wearing his one-piece footie romper all day long).

You can make the process of decorating and furnishing the baby's room and choosing the layette as simple or as complicated as you desire, but the fact remains that the baby's needs are fairly basic . . . initially. Oh yes, you will be shelling out plenty as the years go by—the toys, then tuition—so go easy on the newborn outfits, which your baby grows out of within weeks. Some additional hints:

■ Register for many of these items for your baby shower. Grandparents and other close family members may wish to purchase the "big ticket" baby carriage, for example, and friends will enjoy being able to choose other items you've selected yourself.

■ Borrow from siblings, friends, neighbors, etc. Many people are thrilled to unload baby gear and clothing that are only gently used but taking up space. Added bonus: They've already done the hard work of selection, so you don't have to waste hours wondering which brand, which model, which color, and so forth.

■ Check consignment shops for good prices on gently used items. Since most newborns get merely a month or two of wear out of any one item, the vast majority of consignment store goods are *very* gently used.

The Bare Necessities

Here are the essential items you will want to have on hand from the moment you leave the hospital.

- going-home outfit for baby (although the hospital-issue variety is usually quite serviceable), including cap and blanket
- backward-facing car seat for newborn
- newborn diapers (these are usually marked "NB")
- diaper cream
- wipes
- alcohol swabs for the umbilical cord stump
- petroleum jelly (for diaper rash or to soothe other newborn raw skin spots; also to treat circumcision)
- breast pump (if you are breast-feeding, a pump is essential)
- nursing bras and breast pads
- infant formula, bottles, and nipples (if you are bottle feeding)
- pacifiers (if you choose to use them)
- thermometer

In the early days, your little one may require frequent and quick changes as you get into the rhythm of feeding and diaper changing, so be prepared with at least one weeks' supply of

- kimono-style snap-front shirts (easier to put on than a shirt over baby's head)
- one-piece sleepers/rompers
- sack-style sleepers (for fuss-free middle-of-the-night changing)
- swaddling blankets

The key pieces of "hardware" you'll want to have set up and ready to go in baby's room or sleeping area include:

Changing table and pad. These tables are usually equipped with an easily accessible top drawer to hold diapering essentials and drawers or shelves for outfits.

Bassinet, Moses basket, co-sleeper, or crib. What you choose depends on whether your baby will be sleeping in your room or her own, but initially at least, you will want to have baby close by in a bassinet, basket, or co-sleeper. Be sure to place a good supply of sheets and waterproof mattress covers or pads in the sleeping quarters. Babies are often leaky.

Diaper pail. These really do help contain unpleasant odors, which begin to emit from the diapers especially once baby goes on solid foods.

Rocker or gliding chair. This is a delightful addition to your nursery, particularly if you are breast-feeding (the arm rests will help you maintain optimal nursing position). Make sure the chair's arm is at a comfortable height.

Hard to believe, but you will soon be bathing and shampooing your little one as if you've been doing it all your life. Fortunately, you can do so without too much special equipment—after all, back in the day your mom probably bathed you in the kitchen sink. It's a good idea to have on hand:

- baby wash/baby shampoo
- baby plastic tub (to go in the sink or bath tub)
- baby washcloths
- baby towel or absorbent robe

⚠ **EXPERT TIP:** *Bathe baby from head to toe—not toe to head. You don't want to transfer germs from the nether parts up to the face.*

One last essential is a baby stroller that works with your infant car seat. These "convertible" strollers allow you to simply lock the car seat into place so you and baby can take it on the road and get some much-needed fresh air. (Note: These strollers are generally appropriate for baby's first six months; check the weight limit on your car seat and stroller to be certain.)

Beyond the Bare Necessities

The business of baby accoutrements probably accounts for a good part of many nations' gross domestic product. But do you really need these items? Certainly, there are a few that make life much more pleasant, including:

Burp cloths: For those everyday spit-ups and more, have a couple in the rooms where you and baby spend the most time, along with one for the diaper bag (see page 144). If your baby is a real spitter-upper, have one in every room of the house so you'll always be prepared.

Baby monitor: A blessing and a curse for new parents: Some compare listening to it through the night to being posted on nuclear-missile watch. Who knew babies made so much incidental squawking and random sounds? Monitors are indispensable should the baby's room be situated far from your bedroom or other rooms of the house, and you need to be alert for the next feeding. But sleeping with one by your bedside will have you listening to every breath, cough, and coo. Purchase one but keep the volume low, especially if you want to get some sleep.

SUPPLIES AND DEMANDS: You can categorize purchases for your

(Fig. A)
BARE NECESSITY ITEMS:

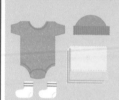
Outfit and Blanket

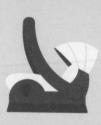
Car Seat

Newborn Diapers

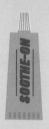
Diaper Cream

Wipes

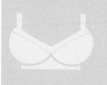
Swabs

Pertroleum Jelly

Breast Pump

Nursing Bras

Bottles

Pacifier

Thermometer

Snap-front Shirts

One-piece Sleeper

Sack-style Sleepers

Swaddling Blanket

newborn from the bare necessities to deferred-purchase plan.

(Fig. B)
BASIC HARDWARE:

1. Changing table
2. Bassinet or crib
3. Diaper pail
4. Rocker or glider

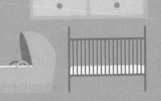
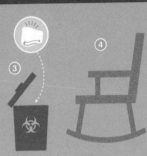

(Fig. C)
BEYOND BARE NECESSITIES:

1. Baby monitor
2. Diaper bag
3. Bottle warmer
4. Baby sling
5. Baby carrier
6. Nursing pillow
7. Burp cloths
8. Baby book library

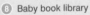

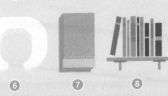

(Fig. D)
DEFERRED ITEMS:

1. Umbrella stroller
2. Jogging stroller
3. High chair
4. Bouncy seat
5. Floor gym

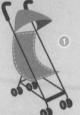
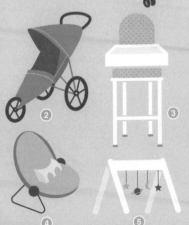

Bottle warmer: Useful if you are doing bottle feeding or a bottle-and-breast combo. But note that running the bottle under the warm tap will also do the trick. Double-check that the size of the warmer is compatible with the type of bottle you are using.

Diaper bag: Yes, you can get by without one, but when the designs today are so chic and ergonomically pleasing, why should you? Just note that you do not need to carry a year's supply of anything in the bag, so keep it small, contained, and easy to carry. Tip: Keep your bag battle ready at all times. If you must get out of the house (to settle the baby with fresh air, for a medical emergency, when running out to meet a friend for coffee at the last minute), you don't want to race around the house like a madwoman tracking down wipes, toys, pacifiers, backup clothes, etc.

Nursing pillow: These come in various designs, and if you're planning to nurse, they can be a major help in positioning you and baby for greatest comfort.

Baby carrier: These front-wearing carriers are wonderful for you and the baby, plus they leave you hands-free for doing chores and other tasks. Baby can face mom until she is old enough to turn around and face front, usually when she has good neck strength. Be careful to place the fulcrum of the straps in the right spot on your back to prevent aches and soreness.

Baby sling: A sling allows for lots of baby-parent contact with minimal hardware and straps. Slings seem to generate less back pain because the weight of the baby is distributed across the parent's shoulders and back.

Library for you and baby: Get a few of the comprehensive baby and parenting books. You may have a thousand minor and major questions, and it's nice to have these handy while you're waiting for a return call from your pediatrician. Start building your baby's library, too, with some classics that you can use for bedtime rituals and more. It is important to read to your baby for language acquisition, and it's a fun activity no matter how old your child is.

Travel crib: Modern travel cribs seem to fold up into astonishingly small packages that are remarkably lightweight and well designed. You can even use this crib around the house to park the baby for a time or, with models that have a changing-table option, for quick diaper changes.

The Deferred-Purchase Plan

Despite what baby-supply retailers may have you believe, there really is no reason to purchase a lot of baby gear before your little one is born—and there are even more items you can simply and intelligently defer until after you know what you really want and need, not to mention what's appropriate for your child.

   Things to get as the months go by include

Umbrella stroller: These are terrific for convenience. They are lightweight and collapsible (usually with one easy motion) and thus are great for storage, airplane rides, or tossing in the trunk of the car or taxi. Most are not meant for children younger than six months (baby's head and neck muscles need to strengthen).

Conventional or jogging stroller: Once baby grows out of the convertible car seat/stroller combo, you can begin to research options for your go-to stroller—the one that will last you through toddlerhood, ideally. Depending on the terrain you typically traverse (off-road jogging trails? city streets?), you can choose from an infinite variety of strollers that fit your needs.

High chair: You won't have to worry about finding the perfect high chair until about the time your baby starts eating solid foods and can sit upright on his own. Safety is obviously the highest priority, so make sure the chair has a five-point harness to buckle him in and that it cannot tip even with the most determined wiggling. The next priority may be how easy it is to clean. High chairs can become unpleasant reservoirs of pooled liquids, food encrustation, and other bodily residues (spit up, drool, leaky diapers, etc.), so look for one that can be thoroughly and conveniently washed.

Bouncy seat: These fabric-covered, lightweight seats are wonderful for entertaining baby (some come equipped with toys and music players), especially when Mom or Dad needs free hands for a moment. They also give baby a chance to change her perspective by sitting more independently.

Floor gym, saucer-style activity chair, swing, and jumper. These are all excellent ways to engage baby's attention while she remains safe and secure. Just make sure to follow the manufacturer's setup instructions.

 JUST FOR DADS: *A few pointers about baby accoutrements:*

■ *Consider roping in a buddy to help assemble items such as the crib and changing table. Make it a male-bonding event: Get a six-pack of beer and chips and then wrestle that pesky crib into existence. Sneaky trick: If you are truly incapable of putting stuff together, serve the chips in small bowls. That way you can keep excusing yourself to get refills. Loiter in the kitchen until your friend hollers for help. Bring lots of food to appease his irritation at being left alone to put together your baby's crib.*

■ *Be sure to tell your partner to get a neutral-looking diaper bag. Skip the toile or pink-bunny-yellow-chicks pattern. If she expects you to help with the schlepping, toting around something more macho will go a long way.*

■ *A properly installed car seat is critical. Make sure you have a professional install it or inspect your work so that you know it's safe. Many fire departments have firefighters who are trained to check for correct installation. Call your local fire station and make an appointment or ask if you can stop by.*

■ *You'll soon realize your life has changed when you end up at the office with pacifiers in your pockets.*

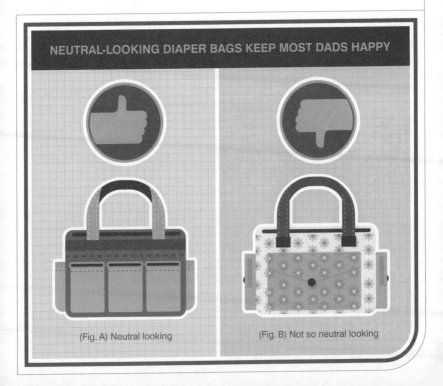

NEUTRAL-LOOKING DIAPER BAGS KEEP MOST DADS HAPPY

(Fig. A) Neutral looking

(Fig. B) Not so neutral looking

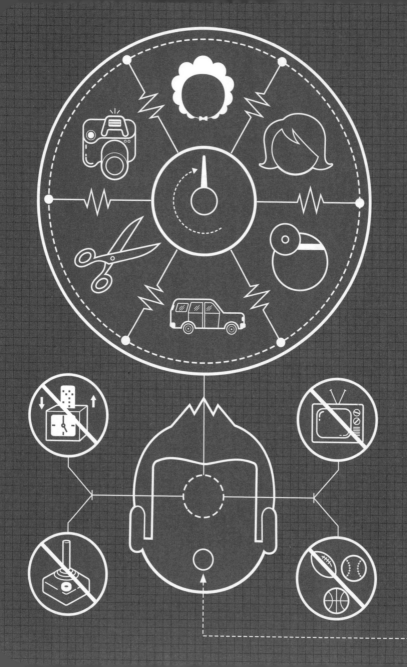

Chapter 6

What Every Expectant Dad Should Know

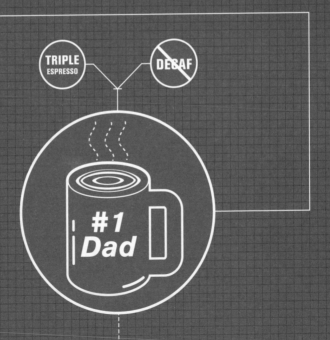

Pregnancy is stressful not just for the expectant mom. Men, too, are affected by the impending change in their lives. The major difference is that men get little to zero sympathy and are expected to soldier on without complaint. But men experience a range of emotional and sometimes physical changes as they take on the role of dad-to-be.

Signs That You Really Are an Expectant Father

Men are often puzzled witnesses to the pregnancy roller-coaster ride. They watch with detached wonder at the eye-rolling panic, screaming, and giddy hilarity as their partners whip around emotional curves, do grueling loop-de-loops, and vomit at the quiet moments. But men have reactions all their own to these new circumstances on the home front.

Repulsion. Pregnancy is supposed to be a beautiful, natural state, but some men might feel uncomfortable with all the changes their partner is experiencing. Watching her tummy undulate and wobble when the baby is kicking might make him think more about horror movies than nature's miracle of life. Also, the leaking, wheezing, gassy, crabby, hungry, snoring, bulky woman with bad skin lying in bed next to you may not be your physical ideal. Men, give yourselves a break and acknowledge that your feelings are okay (just don't share them with her), and remember that your partner will be even more awesome postpartum, when she has returned to her normal self but has become the mother of your child. Some lucky men will even find themselves with a more attractive, curvier postpartum gal.

Provider anxiety. While your pregnant partner is cooing over her latest addition to the layette, you may be feeling a growing weight on your shoulders about providing for the little bundle of joy. Babies ain't cheap, and you and your partner would be advised to map out costs and expenditures. Discussing a budget and collaborating on where to spend and where to save may help manage expectations and also relieve you of the burden of thinking that you are the only one mindful of money matters.

Career anxiety. His and hers. Having a baby can trigger other big life changes:

■ Your partner may want to stop working and become a stay-at-home mom.

■ She may be interested in part-time work or a long maternity leave.

■ Make sure you both know what the other's expectations are for future work.

■ If both partners worked full-time jobs, you will have to reassess your spending if one of you quits. Keep in mind that sometimes daycare or full-time nanny care is as expensive as one full-time salary.

■ Make your calculations and spend time thinking about how to navigate your wishes of raising your child and managing careers and incomes.

■ It may be helpful to establish a tentative five-year plan.

Financial anxieties. You may benefit from airing out your financial concerns if your partner is the main breadwinner.

[1] Remember to have any money discussions only when you are both well rested, willing, and ready.

[2] Set up an appointment with each other for an optimum time and day of the week so that you both are prepared for the discussion.

[3] Use neutral terms; remember, you are a team, not opposing sides. Employ "I" phrases, such as "I am worried that we won't have enough money for the basics if we take our annual splurge vacation." Or "I know it feels like you must have that four-poster princess canopy bed, but she really won't be using it for another three years. Couldn't we just stick with your sister's bassinet for now?"

[4] Keep in mind that decisions do not need to be made all at once, but you would be wise to begin to isolate the issues near the end of the second trimester and decide how you will go about solving them as a team.

Couvade syndrome: This exotic-sounding term is known in medical circles as "sympathetic pregnancy." It occurs when the dad-to-be begins to experience pregnancy symptoms, such as nausea, weight gain, and mood swings, among others. All sorts of psychological and hormonal reasons explain why the expectant dad manifests these symptoms, but so does the simple fact that there may be more goodies around the house (ice cream for two is so much more fun) and that, when one person in a household gets out of sorts, it often triggers the other to feel touchy, too. Dad may be hitting that pleasure center of the brain with tubs of Ben & Jerry's Chubby Hubby ice cream since his sex life has dwindled to nothing. So, watch what you eat and be sure to exercise regularly to clear your head and crank up your metabolism.

Feeling neglected: Many men feel neglected during their partner's pregnancy. If you are one of them, just wait till the baby arrives and then you will know what real neglect is. Seriously, you may feel as though all your partner thinks about is herself and the baby, which is likely true. The first trimester is a real grind, as is the third. Your best bet for attention is during

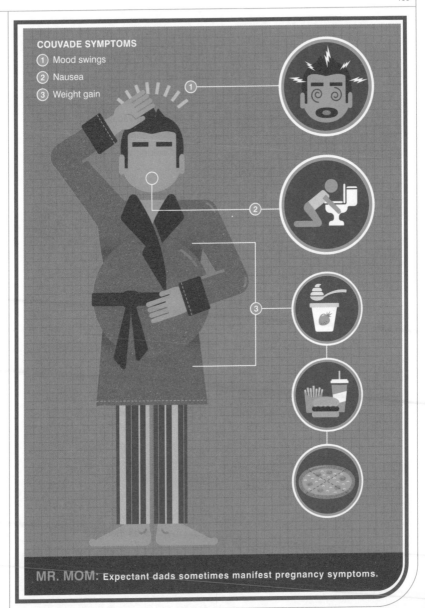

the second trimester. Plan a romantic getaway for that time and take pictures. Or set up dates so that she can nap in advance and prepare herself for some quality time with you.

Feeling like you're walking on egg shells: You may also notice that when she finally does pay attention, you are the target of her irritation: "You still haven't changed the litter box!" Dad, take heed: You do not want to antagonize her and get into a bicker spiral. Just roll with it and acknowledge that she may be crabby because of her physical discomforts and hormonal state. Some things that might help:

[1] Neutralize her anger by being really, really solicitous of her aches and pains. You may find a surprising change of attitude if you offer her a back rub or a cup of herbal tea or do some of her errands. (Though if she has become totally nuts, she may squint sideways at you and wonder, "What's his game? Hmm." But at least then you'll win some time as she quietly contemplates your disconcerting kindness.)

[2] Take a deep breath and tell her how much you admire all the hard work she is doing growing your baby. What woman could resist such gallantry?

[3] Be sincere. A pregnant woman's sarcasm detector is vigilant. If she knows she can go to you for support when feeling low, you will soon become the object of her reawakened affection rather than her scorn.

Planning for Time Off to Spend with Baby

Here's another issue you will want to air out sooner rather than later: How much time, if any, do you plan to spend with your new baby in the first few months after birth?

Your partner will need lots of support when she comes home from the hospital. First-time parents can be panic stricken at the thought of being left alone with a newborn, and if mom is recovering from a C-section or other surgical procedures, she will be even more grateful for an able body to help out.

You, on the other hand, will likely have an irresistible urge to retreat to the safe and predictable haven of work. Your partner knows that. Do not even attempt to make your work sound anywhere close to the realm of her newfound job—especially if you are one of those dads who insists on sleeping through the night because you have to be "fresh for work." Just return home as soon as possible and refrain from making remarks such as, "Wow, it is so great to be able to have an adult conversation that doesn't involve diaper rash, nipple confusion, or umbilical stumps."

Talk to your partner about your vision for those first weeks. Consider:

■ Will your employer want you to use up sick and vacation days before taking unpaid leave?

■ Does your employer have a paternity-leave policy? Some companies provide paid, or partially paid, leaves of varying lengths, and most offer some amount of unpaid leave.

■ Are you eligible for any other form of family leave?

■ Are there more creative ways to take the time off? Perhaps you won't use the leave time in 12 successive weeks but over several months, with partial work weeks over a longer period.

■ It is wise to map out a plan with your employer early and get it in writing so there is no confusion.

Dad and Doc:
Preparing for Prenatal Visits

There are a few appointments and procedures during pregnancy that the expectant dad should plan to attend.

[1] The first prenatal visit to the obstetrician or midwife is one of the most important appointments. You will meet your partner's caregiver, share your family histories, and see the heartbeat (the blinking peanut) on the ultrasound for the first time. You are also invaluable as a second set of ears to catch critical information that your partner may miss.

Important tip: Be sure to bring a pen and paper to take notes. Better yet, come prepared with your own written list of questions and concerns. This visit will be over quickly, so it is helpful to have your questions at the ready.

[2] Appointments are typically once a month for normal pregnancies in the first two trimesters and into the third. You will want to attend the appointment when you get to listen to the baby's heartbeat for the first time. Make sure the caregiver tells you when that one will happen; usually it occurs at the 12-week visit. This appointment is also a good time to review what prenatal testing is appropriate for your partner and to have questions answered while all parties are present.

[3] Partners will want to attend any invasive-testing appointments (such as CVS or amniocentesis) to provide moral support when the mom-to-be may feel particularly anxious. Your mere presence will help her relax.

[4] Don't miss the big anatomy ultrasound at week 19 or 20, when you can learn the sex of your baby. Most partners also simply love to watch their baby on the ultrasound, and at this stage you may see some real fetal activity, including thumb sucking and arm and leg movements. You will also be treated to views of baby's brain, kidney, heart chambers, bladder, and spine.

Important tip: If you do not wish to learn the sex of your baby, be sure to share your preference with your doctor, attending nurses, and the ultrasound technician. They should note it in your file for the duration of the pregnancy and take appropriate care not to reveal the gender.

[5] Many men do not attend prenatal appointments until they are weekly, near the end of the pregnancy. These last few appointments can be helpful for reviewing the signs of labor and ways to time contractions. The doctor may also review problems that can develop near the end of the pregnancy, such as blood pressure issues, decreased fetal movements, and bleeding. Again, having a second pair of ears to hear precautions and restrictions can be advantageous.

DOC TALK: The anatomy ultrasound at 19–20 weeks is a must for dads. For many men, up to this point the pregnancy has been abstract. They are downright perplexed by the severity of symptoms in the first half of pregnancy. Many a father has pulled me to the side with such comments as: "C'mon, doc, how can that little blip on the ultrasound that's no bigger than my toe be making my wife sick?" Of course, in the early stages many men are having a blast. They have their built-in designated driver on evenings out and can watch sports while Mom zonks out on the couch. But after the anatomy ultrasound, I see the look in their eyes as they realize what Mom has been going through and that their child is really growing inside her.

A Birthing Coach's Motto: Be Prepared

You should plan for several key logistics before those first labor contractions. Having a plan will ease your mind about your roles as labor coach and designated emergency chauffeur.

[1] Attend a childbirth class. Your partner is doing all the work, but it doesn't hurt to get some facts about what will be happening to her and the baby during labor and delivery. A comprehensive childbirth class will help you understand the labor stages and enhance your role as a useful birth coach. Remember, your partner's mind may become a little inwardly focused as contractions begin, so learning the basics about how to time them will help you determine when to get her to the hospital or birthing center.

You'll also learn coaching techniques to help Mom with active labor, including how to:

■ encourage her to shift positions, squat, or walk around to work through contractions.

■ apply the breathing techniques you both learned in class.

■ massage her or brush her hair to help her relax.

■ focus her mind on helpful, calming images or play music that will help soothe or inspire her.

■ help her into the shower to relieve pain and tension.

Be sure to write down the techniques that your partner prefers, so you can refer to them when the birthing process starts. Otherwise, your mind may go blank when you need to do *something*.

VEHICULAR NAVIGATION: Know the lay of the land before the big day.

HOME

COUNTY HOSPITAL

ROUTES TO HOSPITAL

- - - SHORTER DISTANCE
MORE DELAYS

- - - LONGER DISTANCE
FEWER DELAYS

[2] Take a hospital tour. It will help you and your partner visualize where the birth will take place. It is critical that you note the location of

- the main entrance
- the after-hours entrance
- long-term parking
- valet parking
- places to double park in case of a quick drop-off
- emergency room entrance

You should also note the location of pay phones; cafeteria or vending machines; maternity waiting room; and nursery. Find out the hospital's security measures and the system the staff uses to match newborns to parents (often with ID bracelets). You may also register with the hospital now (which will save time should baby be in a rush to come out).

[3] Plan your route to the hospital. Always keep the gas tank filled as the pregnancy comes to term (at week 37). Rehearse the route, noting new construction and potential roadwork delays. Have alternate routes mapped out in case of heavy traffic or unexpected road closings. Make sure you have money or a remote toll pass if you need to use toll roads.

[4] Plan for childcare contingencies. If you have older children, arrange for childcare during your time at the hospital. If you do not want to bring the child with you for the birth, figure out scenarios for different times and days of the week. You may even want to pack a bag for your older children if they will not be attending the birth. Fill it with nonperishable snacks, books, extra clothes and PJs, and any other items that would help your children or the babysitter while you're at the hospital. Leave it by the door so it's ready to go when you are.

[5] Get your camera ready and packed. Load film or charge the battery. Pack a disposable camera as a back-up. Remember to ask a nurse to take a photo of the happy new family after baby's arrival.

How to Be the Best Birth Coach You Can Be

Fortunately for you, doctors, nurses, or a midwife or doula (or some combination thereof) will be around to support your partner during delivery. These trained professionals have medical expertise and will guide her exertions. You are a supplemental, yet essential, support. Men are often a little intimidated by the physical rigors their partners must undergo and how they get through it. All that panting, moaning, sweating, and shaking is intense. Just go with the flow and try to anticipate what she might need.

You are uniquely positioned to be your partner's best advocate:

■ If she is having issues with a nurse, you can do the talking and request a new one.

■ If there are overly zealous residents trying to practice internal exam checks, you can put a stop to it.

■ Cultivate the ideal environment so that your partner can focus on her hard work birthing the baby.

■ Though you may be surprised at the intensity of labor, you know your partner best and may know better than anyone what might give her comfort and relief.

■ Don't tell her things that you aren't qualified to know. But if you think it will help, tell her what you do know: How impressive she is; that the nurses say

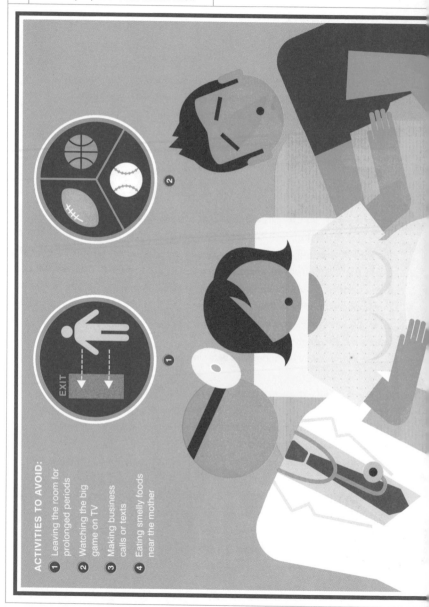

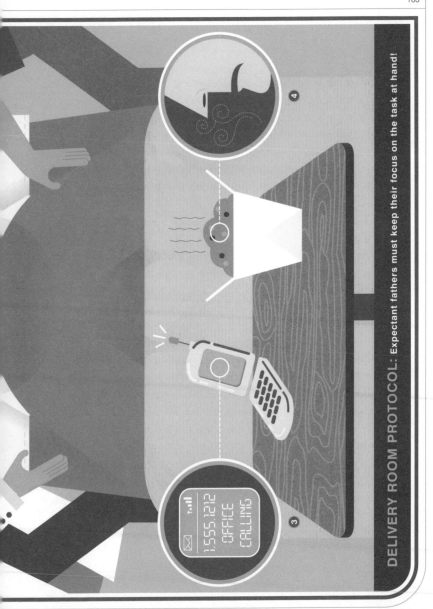

DELIVERY ROOM PROTOCOL: Expectant fathers must keep their focus on the task at hand!

she's doing all the right things; that the doctor says everything is progressing wonderfully; that you are proud of her.

■ Know the times when she needs you to be quiet. You are helping just by being a familiar, reassuring presence during her efforts.

■ If she starts vomiting, check with the nurse and then relay that the nurse says it's a good sign of the body's transition. If she is shaking, check what that means with the nurse and then reassure her that the nurse says it means that labor is progressing.

■ Even simply holding her hand and letting her squeeze it may be just what she needs.

■ Remember your childbirth-class training and, if you sense she is receptive, suggest things she can do to ease her pain. Don't be surprised if she seems to tune you out, but look for the spaces between contractions when she can speak, and you may get an affirmative to one of your suggestions. There may also be a time during labor when she shoos you away. That is natural and should be accepted gracefully.

■ Don't leave the room for unexplained reasons or long periods. Don't eat smelly food near her. Don't watch the game on television (even if she says it's okay, it is not), and don't make business phone calls, send text messages, or in any way seem distracted from the task at hand. Though she may not want to talk to you, she wants to have you ready and receptive when she changes her mind.

DOC TALK: *Labor and delivery are incredibly dynamic processes that can change instantaneously. Emergencies arise in the blink of an eye, and it is imperative that a couple feels comfortable and confident in their provider's advice and assessment. In addition, it can be a very helpless feeling to watch the person you love experiencing pain at the extremes of human endurance. In these circumstances, partners can be emotional, demanding* *pain relief when oftentimes the patient herself is refusing—a perfect example of why communication is so vital during the prenatal course as well as during labor (not to mention in child rearing).*

Cutting the Umbilical Cord

After your partner delivers the baby, your practitioner will place two clamps on the umbilical cord and offer the dad the chance to cut it. When to do the cutting will depend on maternal wishes, location of birth, and whether you are banking the cord blood. In some cultures, leaving the cord intact for a while after the birth is desirable and respectful. If you are storing the blood, the cord blood will be extracted at this time.

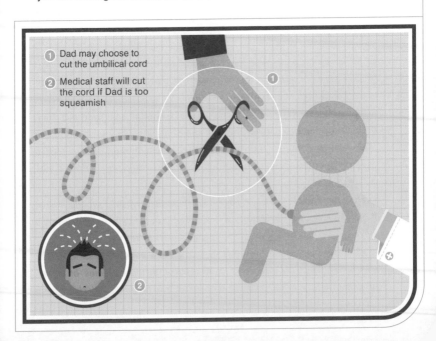

1 Dad may choose to cut the umbilical cord

2 Medical staff will cut the cord if Dad is too squeamish

Be prepared: This rite of passage can often be quite powerful emotionally, though some dads are just too darn squeamish and don't want to do it. Feel free to speak up. The medical staff would rather do it themselves than have you pass out.

How to Perform an Emergency Delivery

Keep in mind that a dramatic delivery means your child will be forever blessed with an awesome story for every future birthday party. ("Well, my mom and dad mistimed the contractions and had to pull over onto the shoulder of the bridge during the blizzard, when . . .")

Next, remember that birth has been happening for millions of years without monitors, sterile equipment, or fancy instruments, so do not panic. Here's what you need to know and do if the baby is coming and you haven't reached a medical center:

■ Pull over and call emergency services.

■ Have Mom lie down on the backseat and place a clean sheet or towel under her bottom (a shirt will do).

■ If possible, clean your hands and get ready to catch.

■ Once the head emerges, the rest of the body usually comes quickly afterward. Sometimes gentle traction may be needed. That can be accomplished by placing one's hands under the baby's armpits and pulling gently.

■ Wrap the baby in a shirt or towel for warmth.

■ Hand the baby off to Mom.

Note: If a baby is born quickly, he may not realize that he needs to start breathing on his own. If the baby appears blue or limp and is not vigorously crying, you may need to stimulate him by rubbing the soles of his

feet or rubbing up and down his spine. If help has still not arrived, you may
need to cut the umbilical cord:

■ Note that there are typically three blood vessels in the cord, so it must be clamped in two places to prevent blood loss from baby and Mom.

■ Take a shoelace (or string, cloth strips, or dental floss) and tie a tight knot in two places on the cord about 1 inch (2.5 cm) apart.

■ Use a clean pocketknife or scissors to cut the cord between the knots.

■ If help has still not arrived, you may need to deliver the placenta.

■ Remember that the umbilical cord will still be coming from Mom's vagina with a little knot at the end. This portion of cord is still attached to the placenta.

■ You do not need to pull on the cord. The placenta will deliver itself, usually within 30 minutes after the baby is born.

■ If it does come out on its own, you will usually see a large gush of blood and clots. Do not panic. Mom's body is still sending a large quantity of blood to the uterus—it takes a moment to realize that the baby is no longer attached.

■ Usually, the uterus will contract quickly after the placenta comes out. As the uterine muscle contracts and squeezes, it decreases this bleeding substantially.

■ If blood continues to come out heavily, massage the uterus by rubbing Mom's belly vigorously. (You can usually feel the uterus as a firm ball between the pubic bone and belly button.) This massage reminds the uterus that it must contract.

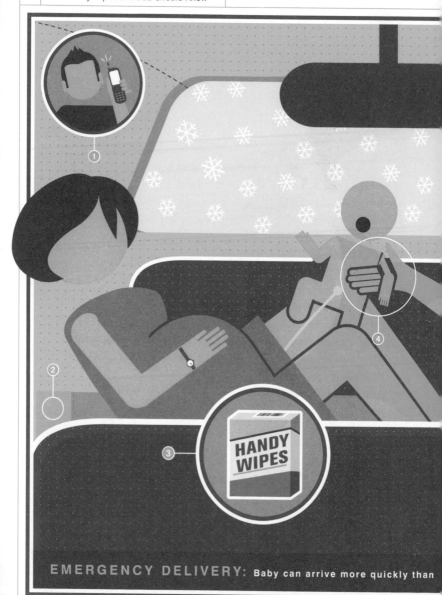

EMERGENCY DELIVERY: Baby can arrive more quickly than

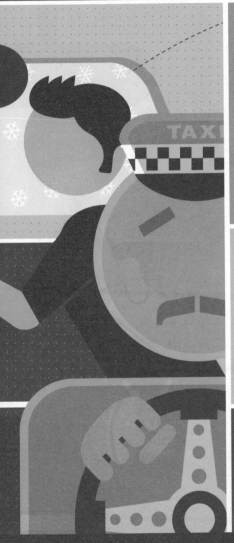

1. Call emergency services.

2. Have Mom lie down on the back-seat and place a clean sheet or towel under her bottom.

3. If possible, clean your hands and get ready to catch.

4. Once head emerges, your assistance pulling may be needed. Try placing hand under the baby's armpit and pull gently.

5. Wrap baby in shirt or towel for warmth.

6. Hand the baby off to Mom.

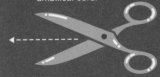

⚠️ If help has still not arrived, you may need to cut the umbilical cord.

expected so be prepared. Remember your birthing classes, and don't panic!

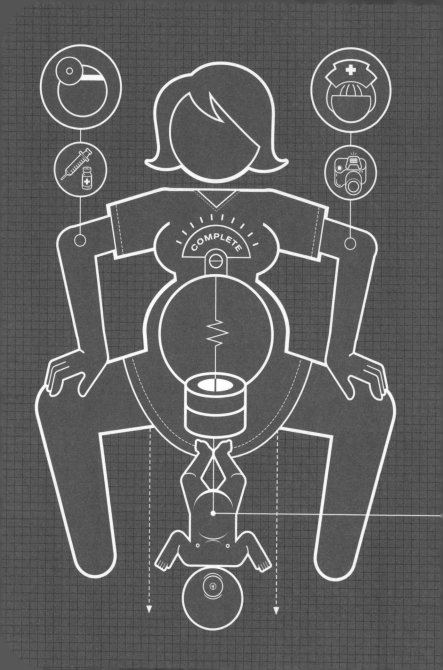

Chapter 7

The Grand Finale— Here Comes Baby

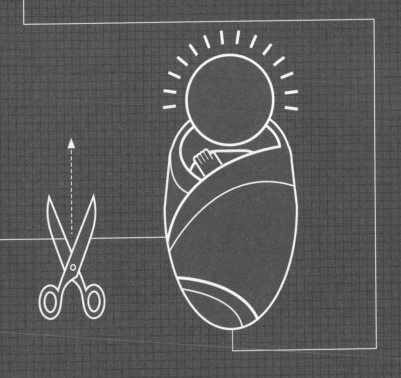

Childbirth is both an epic and an everyday occurrence: It's a fascinating combination of the extraordinary and the routine. First-timers wonder—and know they don't know, no matter how many episodes of some maternity show they watch on TV—what their first time will be like. Am I gonna make it? (You will.) Will I be a screamer or quiet and intent? (Think back about 40 weeks ago and remember how all this got started . . .) Could it really be as hard as all those stories I've heard? (For most women, no.) Can I stay relaxed and comfortable and have a terrific, empowering birth experience? (You will soon find out.)

Moms are addicted to sharing their birth stories, so by the time you hit your ninth month, you will have heard all the variations on this theme. And yes, we all love to hear the ones where the woman stays calm, in touch with her primal birthing self, and feels fantastic and elated by the process. But there is nothing as reassuring as hearing your self-confessed pain-adverse, scaredy cat, prima donna friend tell you: "Heck, if I can do it, anyone can." Then you think, "She's right. She is a wimp. Certainly more of a crybaby than I am. I can do this!" Ahh, your spirits brighten. It also helps to reprioritize your concerns when experienced moms point out in their hard-as-nails, gravely voice of experience: "Hell, childbirth was nothing. Just wait until you try breast-feeding."

As your due date approaches, stop and notice all the people walking around in the world and try to imagine all the women who pushed these people out of their bodies. It's sort of a funny experiment to scan the populace and recast everyone in their infantile state. This mental exercise may help you realize that our bodies are built for this and know what to do. And it's almost your turn. So stay relaxed and calm and enjoy this special time. Savor the joy of having a magic little person growing inside your womb. You will realize later how brief a time it really is.

So get ready for show time: Here comes baby!

Signs That Labor Is Near

You've seen it in countless movies: The sudden, dawning realization that the pregnant mom must get to the hospital STAT! The mom becomes an insult-spewing harridan ("*You* did this to me!"). She's doubled-over in agony, pausing in her moaning only to shower more abuse on her hapless and panic-stricken husband, who suddenly forgets everything he learned in Lamaze class, overlooks the bag intended for the hospital, and invariably steers the car directly into a traffic jam, where he is forced to deliver the baby himself.

The truth is, however, most couples have more than sufficient warning that labor is about to happen in earnest. No one knows precisely what triggers labor, but several clues suggest that it is approaching fast. Here are some signposts that tell you it is time to get the bag—and the mom—in the car.

Due date: Statistically speaking, the due date is a marker of when your baby will likely be ready to emerge. Most women give birth sometime between week 37 and week 42. Though most women do not give birth on their due date, it is a useful milestone for gauging your preparedness. When you see your due date looming on the calendar, you should begin to pay attention to your body for its signals. Be prepared for a surge of excitement (tinged with panic) the moment the calendar date turns to the birth month. It won't be long now!

"Lightening": Lightening, or when the baby "drops," occurs when the baby engages into the pelvic cradle. As she moves lower (head first) into your pelvis, she is preparing for her trip down the birth canal. However, this symptom is a bit of a red herring for those women who experience lightening days or weeks before labor, and some women's babies never engage until active labor. But as you get more intense and frequent Braxton Hicks contractions, they will push the baby lower into the pelvis, which will put pressure on the cervix and start to soften and thin it.

Loose stools: Hormonal changes triggered by prostaglandins before labor can produce loose stools. It makes sense: Your body is evacuating the colon to make room for the baby to pass through the pelvic area.

"Water" breaks: Sometimes the amniotic sac is referred to by the strangely biblical-sounding term "bag of waters." When the bag of waters is punctured (whether in the natural course of labor or by your physician), you will be giving birth within 24 to 48 hours. Most doctors do not want to risk infection and wait beyond 24 hours after the baby's environment has been opened to the greater world, especially if the baby is at "term."

If That Bag of Water Breaks

When your amniotic sac breaks, it can create quite a splash—and you may not be in control of just where and when that happens. In the third trimester, the amniotic sac contains about one liter of amniotic fluid and has been providing baby with a cushiony environment throughout his stay in the womb. (Try pouring a liter bottle of water on the floor to get a sense of the spill.) Keep in mind:

■ Some women experience just a small leak.

■ The amniotic sac will continue to leak even after your water breaks, since your body will continue to produce the fluid.

■ Some women do not experience their water "breaking" at all, so to help labor progress the physician will perform an amniotomy by puncturing the sac with a long plastic hook.

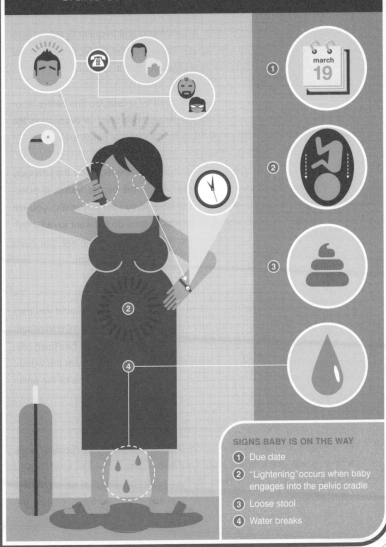

SIGNS OF CHILD DELIVERY INITIALIZATION

SIGNS BABY IS ON THE WAY

1. Due date
2. "Lightening" occurs when baby engages into the pelvic cradle
3. Loose stool
4. Water breaks

■ The fluid should be clearish. If it is darker (green, brown, yellow), it could indicate that your baby has passed his first stool, called meconium, in utero. That is sometimes an indicator of fetal stress. Call your doctor immediately.

DOC TALK: *It is completely normal to experience increased vaginal discharge later in pregnancy. About 10 to 20 percent of women have enough discharge at this stage that they have to wear a feminine pad all the time. Blood flow to the vagina and cervix increases in the third trimester, and the vaginal secretion glands are in overdrive. It can be confusing to know whether you are simply producing more discharge or whether your water has indeed broken: I tell patients that if you feel wet, dry yourself off and walk around. If the water continues to run down your leg, call your doc.*

Spotting, or "bloody show": Bleeding before labor occurs due to changes in your cervix as it prepares to open. As contractions ripen and soften the cervix, capillaries within start to bleed, producing the spotting. As the contractions intesify, you may see some "bloody show" (a quite dramatic term for an ultimately benign symptom). Any stress on the cervix may also cause small amounts of bleeding (from exercise, intercourse, or even straining during a bowel or bladder movement). If you are unsure whether the bleeding is normal, call your doctor.

Mucus plug disengages: As the cervix softens and begins to dilate, the mucus in the cervical canal will often come out. This may be a slow release of mucus discharge, or the "plug" may come out in a knotlike, thick bundle. Until now, the mucus has been acting as a barrier on the cervix, and it is continually produced, especially around the time of delivery. Though the discharge of this mucus is not a sign of impending labor—some women pass the mucus plug and stay pregnant for weeks—it is typically a sign that things are starting to happen.

Back pain: This discomfort can occur if the baby is facing out rather than facing your spine. If the baby does not turn toward your spine, you will have more pain. You may also feel back pain from the baby's head pressing on your spine as contractions begin.

Contractions: Braxton Hicks contractions are the warm-up for the real thing. These contractions may stop and start a few times, and they often stop when you are more active (while walking, for example). Early labor pains will be erratic in intensity and frequency: Some are so strong they take your breath away, and others feel like cramps. Some are 3–5 minutes apart, and some are 10–15 minutes apart. If the doctor can have a 15-minute conversation with you about whether or not you are in labor and you don't pause during your contractions, then it is probably a false alarm.

Get to Know Your Contractions

At the outset of labor, you may experience a contraction once every 20 minutes, each lasting about 30 seconds.

■ Early contractions can feel like menstrual cramps with radiating pain. Your uterine muscle is beginning its work to open the cervix to its full 10 centimeters.

■ Later contractions escalate off the scale of severe menstrual cramps to a level you never knew possible.

■ You will know it is the real thing when the contractions intensify and the uterine muscle gets into a regular rhythm of hard contractions every three to five minutes.

There are no rules about when you need to be at the hospital. But if the contractions are five minutes apart for an hour and are stopping you in your tracks, no one would laugh at you for showing up at the maternity ward. Arrange a game plan with your practitioner that factors in travel time to the hospital.

■ If you live near the hospital, you may need to wait only until the contractions are five minutes apart for an hour before you call and notify the doctor that you are leaving your house and headed her way.

■ If you live 45 minutes from the hospital, you will want to leave with your contractions still further apart.

Talk it over ahead of time so that you are not in a panic when you go into labor. Remember that once true labor starts, most women dilate on average one to two centimeters per hour. So you could calculate having six to eight hours before you even get to the pushing stage. (But if, on your last office visit, you were already four centimeters dilated, you will want to err on the side of an earlier arrival at the hospital.)

⊕ *DOC TALK: I tell expectant parents, especially first-time moms, that we expect a few false alarms. My wife is an ob-gyn, and she made me take her to the hospital three or four times with each of our three children with false alarms! If she can't figure it out, who can? I always tell patients that I would much prefer them to come in and get checked—and if it's a false call go home—than to have them undergo a roadside delivery.*

Timing Is Everything

How do you time contractions? There are two ways. Just be consistent in the method so that you will be aware of their progression.

Method 1

[1] Note when the contraction begins and how long it lasts (for example, 30 seconds to one minute).

[2] Then note when the following contraction begins. If the next one does not occur for nine minutes, then your contractions are ten minutes apart.

[3] Things can be a bit fuzzy when contractions start happening close together. Remember to time from the start of one to the start of the next.

[4] If the contraction begins and lasts one full minute and then you get only three minutes off before the next one, your contractions are now four minutes apart. When they get this close, it may be hard to focus on your watch. Definitely ask someone on your birthing team to begin timing them for you.

Method 2

Same as above, but with this method you will time your contractions from the *end* of one contraction to the *end* of the next.

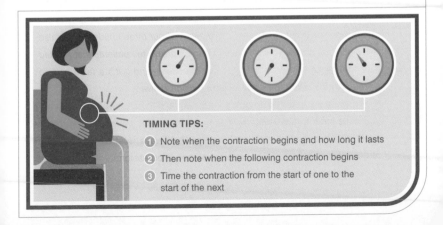

TIMING TIPS:

1. Note when the contraction begins and how long it lasts
2. Then note when the following contraction begins
3. Time the contraction from the start of one to the start of the next

Arriving at the Hospital or Birthing Center

Now that the contractions have started in earnest, it's time to check in to your hospital or birthing center. Just note that some babies don't want to waste time on registration formalities in their hurry to make their grand debut!

The check-in process will vary, but once you have arrived there are some fairly typical procedures. Ask your caregiver if you can preregister at the hospital to get the official stuff (registering insurance, signed consent forms, emergency contact information) out of the way before being admitted. Some obstetrical practices have you all squared away by your second or third appointment. Your records should also be sent to the hospital ahead of time, along with your lab work and pertinent information, just in case of an emergency. When the transfer of medical information happens can vary from place to place, so if you are unsure of the status, ask your doctor.

■ Upon arriving at the maternity ward, you will likely be asked to change into a hospital gown. The birth process is a messy one, so you may even go through one or two.

■ A nurse will check your vital signs (blood pressure, heart rate, temperature, and lungs).

■ You may be asked to give a urine or blood sample.

■ You will be asked how frequent your contractions are and for how long you have been experiencing them. You will also want to inform the nurse if your water has broken and how long ago that happened. They will inquire about the history of your pregnancy and any information on complications or preexisting medical conditions.

■ You will have a pelvic exam to see to what degree your cervix is dilated and effaced.

■ You and the baby may be hooked up for electronic fetal monitoring. Some women request to have monitoring assessed intermittently (rather than continuously) so that their movement is not restricted by leads connected to the machines. The device monitors your baby's heart rate as well as the duration of your contractions to see how baby is tolerating labor.

■ You may receive an intravenous (IV) catheter as a precaution should you require anesthesia, pain relief, fluids, etc. If you are being induced, you will receive medicines (Pitocin) this way. Also, if you have group B strep you will receive antibiotics through the IV during delivery.

⊕ *DOC TALK: Parents often have birth plans, but I ask them to consider them as birth preferences. You cannot control babies and how they will tolerate the birth process. Stay flexible. If you are focused on a natural birth but the baby isn't progressing, sometimes Pitocin will be needed to strengthen contractions. Or if a baby is experiencing distress, sometimes it is safer to be in bed and have continuous monitoring. At these moments it is vital to trust your caregiver to recommend what is safest for you and your baby.*

⚲ *EXPERT TIP: Don't start your phone tree to inform friends and family that you have arrived at the hospital and are giving birth until you are told by your doctor that you are staying. Many moms are turned away and told to return later if they are not far enough along in labor—or if they are experiencing false labor.*

Joining the Labor Force

Once you have been checked in and are garbed in your hospital gown, you will go to the labor and delivery room. If you are at a birthing center or in a birthing suite, you will remain in this room for the whole process. Here's a rundown of what to expect in the hours ahead:

■ The typical length of labor for first-timers is about 10 hours. That breaks down to about 9½ hours for the first stage of labor, 30 minutes for the second, and about 5 minutes for the third stage (see below).

■ The outside norm for first-timers can take 25+ hours for the first stage, 1–2 to two hours for pushing, and 30 minutes to deliver the placenta.

■ It is fairly typical that second-timers will go faster (first stage around 7–8 hours, second stage approximately 8 minutes, and third stage approximately 5 minutes). The reason for speedier delivery the second time around is that once the cervix has dilated from a previous birth, it responds more readily to the signals of labor and has greater elasticity from already being stretched.

Stage 1

This stage is what most people think of as "labor," though it is only one-third of the process. That's because it's the longest phase, and it encompasses three subphases, during which the cervix is dilating: early, with 0–3 centimeter dilation; active, with 3–7 centimeter dilation; and transition, with 7–10 centimeter dilation.

Early labor

Many healthy women in the low-risk category go about their normal activities and remain home during the early stage of labor, when the cervix is softening and thinning.

How you'll feel: You'll have irregular contractions that range from breath-taking to just a bit crampy. This can be a confusing time because it can last for 12–24 hours before the contractions fall into a pattern of active labor. Ease your discomfort with a hot shower or have your partner massage your lower back or hips.

Active labor

By the time active labor begins, you will want to be at the hospital or birthing center, where you will be checked intermittently to make sure the cervix is dilating.

How you'll feel: Your body is releasing endorphins during this process, as a natural pain reliever, but now is the time you can also opt for medicinal pain relief (see "Pain Management 101," page 190). Don't wait until the transition phase to put in your request for the epidural or it may be too late. You may experience shakes and vomiting as a result of the profound exertion your body is experiencing to contract the huge uterine muscle three to five minutes for hours on end.

Transition

At their most intense, contractions can occur every two minutes, and toward the end of the transition phase contractions will last 90 seconds. That gives Mom only 30 seconds of recovery time before the next one. (Now is when most men concede there is no way they could ever, ever birth a baby. You are astonishing your man!)

How you'll feel: At least transition is the shortest part of labor. Most moms will be extremely focused and direct about what works for relief and what does not during this intense time. Labor coaches, be prepared! If you are doing labor naturally, you will need to rely on the relaxation techniques you've been working on for the last few weeks to get through.

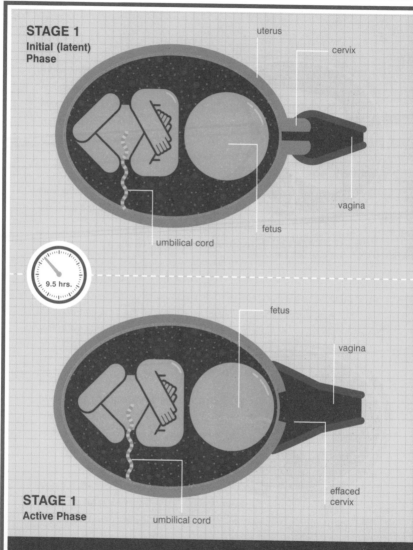

STAGE 1
Initial (latent) Phase

uterus

cervix

vagina

fetus

umbilical cord

9.5 hrs.

fetus

vagina

STAGE 1
Active Phase

umbilical cord

effaced cervix

THE THREE STAGES OF LABOR: Typical length of labor for first-timers is

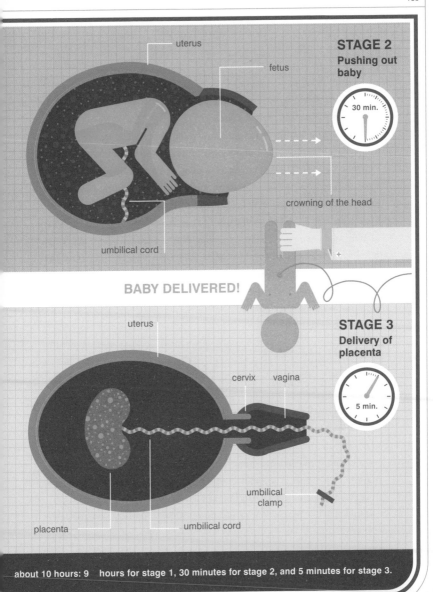

uterus

fetus

STAGE 2
Pushing out baby

30 min.

crowning of the head

umbilical cord

BABY DELIVERED!

uterus

STAGE 3
Delivery of placenta

5 min.

cervix

vagina

umbilical clamp

placenta

umbilical cord

about 10 hours: 9 hours for stage 1, 30 minutes for stage 2, and 5 minutes for stage 3.

Stage 2

Stage 2 is when the cervix is fully dilated, and Mom pushes the baby down and out of the vaginal canal.

How you'll feel: There is frequently a short period of rest from stage 1 to stage 2 before you feel an urge to push. Your practitioner will tell you when you're fully dilated and it's okay to do so safely. Contractions slow during this phase, and some moms are so tired they even doze between pushes. You will feel intense rectal pressure as the baby moves farther down the birth canal. (Many women do indeed pass stool at this point, which means you're pushing the "right" way.) When the baby's head crowns out of the vagina, there can be a burning sensation just before or as the head crests the outer rim that is sometimes called the "ring of fire." Once the head is out, the rest of the baby typically slips out easily.

Stage 3

This stage is the delivery of the placenta, which you may not even notice because at this point you are holding or breast-feeding your baby or are still a bit numb from pain medication. The afterbirth typically occurs within 20 minutes of the baby's arrival. Your practitioner will examine the placenta and make sure no debris or clots were left behind by sweeping his hand around your uterus and removing any found material. This part is uncomfortable but necessary. Debris left behind could cause excess bleeding and infection.

How you'll feel: Woozy. Elated. Sore. Relieved. Exhausted. Congratulations, Mom, you did it! And now you can gaze upon your little bundle. She may be a red-faced screaming bundle, barely opening her eyes, but she's all yours, at least for the next 18 years.

What Does a Baby Look Like at Birth?

First of all, all those "newborn" babies you see on television and in movies are just acting. They are usually several months old by the time their agents score them that sitcom or film deal. No casting director would ever put a real newborn on the silver screen. They just aren't camera ready. Here's why:

■ Childbirth can create quite a mess, with all that amniotic fluid, greasy vernix, maternal poop and pee, and lots and lots of blood (not just the dribs and drabs of a paper cut, but flowing, copious amounts of blood). So baby is often quite a sight upon arrival.

■ Babies' heads are typically cone-shaped when they are first born. That is because the bones of an infant's skull are soft and pliable, allowing baby to squeeze through the birth canal. But don't worry, the head will round itself out. (In the meantime, just put one of those cute newborn caps on baby.)

■ Many babies have substantial bruising of the face, head, and body from the traumatic passage through the birth canal. Noses can look squashed for a day or two.

■ Eyes and genitalia are often swollen initially.

■ The skin can be saggy if the baby is post date.

■ The skin can be dry, blotchy, and rashy.

■ Babies can have a variety of permanent or temporary marks on their skin. "Angel kisses," or salmon patches, are clusters of blood vessels that usually appear on the forehead and fade with time. "Stork bites" are blood vessel clusters that often appear on the nape of the neck and may not fade. Mongolian spots, more common among dark-skinned babies, usually fade in time.

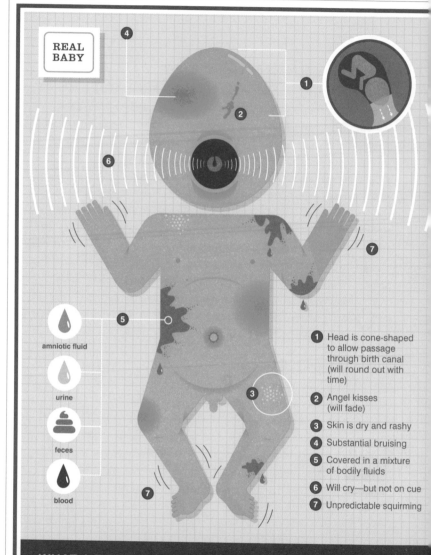

REAL BABY

1. Head is cone-shaped to allow passage through birth canal (will round out with time)

2. Angel kisses (will fade)

3. Skin is dry and rashy

4. Substantial bruising

5. Covered in a mixture of bodily fluids

6. Will cry—but not on cue

7. Unpredictable squirming

amniotic fluid

urine

feces

blood

WHAT A BABY LOOKS LIKE AT BIRTH: Unlike "TV babies," real babies

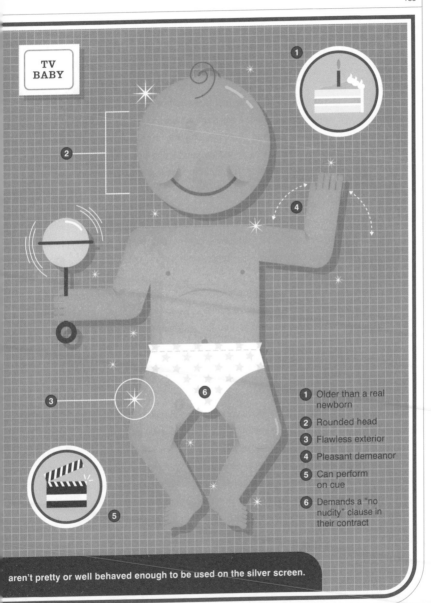

TV BABY

1 Older than a real newborn
2 Rounded head
3 Flawless exterior
4 Pleasant demeanor
5 Can perform on cue
6 Demands a "no nudity" clause in their contract

aren't pretty or well behaved enough to be used on the silver screen.

Pain Management 101

When you're in labor, you may feel overwhelmed by the degree of pain—and the looming thought that it will get a lot worse before it gets better. Now is time for grunting, panting, vomiting, shaking, moaning, and sweating. It's all good! Everyone in the room will be supporting you and your hard work. Here are pain-relief methods that you can employ at home or at the hospital, with medical staff or with your midwife or doula.

Stay at home as long as possible. Doing so will allow you the freedom to move around more and use your own facilities during this early phase. You can sit on a birthing ball, shower, do squats, walk around, listen to music, and eat.

Distract yourself. Focus on photographs of comforting images (beloved pets, children, favorite places or scenes); listen to music; or have your partner distract you by quizzing you on the state capitals.

Breathe. Breathe in through the nose when a contraction begins and out through the mouth as you ride its crest.

Get your free massage. Have your birth coach relieve back labor with a lower back and hip massage, using deep pressure strokes in circular motions; working the spot in the small of your back with a slight upward movement and pressure; applying pressure to either side of your hips; or encircling your belly from underneath it and lifting gently upward. Tennis balls can also be used to soothe and relax tight muscles. Don't forget to relax built-up tension in neck and shoulders—even facial muscles can be massaged to release tension.

Use heat, cold, and moisture. Apply (or have your partner apply) a cool, damp washcloth to your forehead or a hot cloth to your lower back. Doulas swear by this home remedy: Place rice in a long sock and heat it in a microwave or cool it in the freezer; apply to wherever it offers relief. (Even a cold soda can from a vending machine can offer improvised relief.) A warm shower is also incredibly relaxing; bring your birthing ball in the shower and sit on it while the water beats down on you.

Change positions. Let gravity help your body move the baby into the best position. If someone forced you to have your baby in a field, you would probably squat the baby out while leaning against a tree or be on all fours, so feel free to be creative:

■ Squatting will help you widen your pelvis and propel the baby downward.
■ Getting down on hands and knees may relieve pressure on your back.
■ Sometimes hanging between your partner's thighs with your arms hooked over his legs can supply relief.
■ While standing, try draping yourself against your partner for support while allowing your lower back muscles to stretch, or hang onto a bar or knotted sheet secured over a door while squatting and swaying side to side.
■ Immerse yourself in a birthing pool filled with warm, relaxing water.
■ Try lying sideways (avoid being flat on your back), rocking in a rocker, or sitting on the toilet if it feels good.

Get Me the Meds!

You may choose to ask your physician to help with pain-relief medication during labor, and there are some very good reasons to do so:

■ Pain medications can reduce stress and fear, both of which inhibit the birth process.

■ They can help you conserve your energy for when it comes time to push out the baby.

■ If labor has been induced, medicine can relieve the dramatic contractions.

Here is a breakdown of the medicines you can take and their effects:

Narcotic morphine: Narcotics are often used in early labor. *Upside*: They take the edge off contractions but do not affect muscular function, so you can still be up and walking if you choose. *Downside*: Narcotics cross the placenta and can make the baby sleepy; she may then have a more difficult transition from the womb.

Epidural anesthetic: This regional block affects the nerves that innervate the uterus as they leave the spinal column; the epidural is like an IV catheter that goes in the back. *Upside*: It can stay in place for a long time and be adjusted for more or less pain relief. *Downside*: It affects muscle control, so you cannot get out of bed to walk around, find more productive birthing positions, or use the bathroom.

DOC TALK: I remind patients that the epidural is very safe, but it may still have complications. Patients who may not qualify are those who have had previous spinal surgery or those with bleeding disorders. I have my patients consult with our anesthesia department early in the third trimester so that everyone is on the same page and there are no questions on the big day. That is something I recommend all patients address with their doctors long before the baby comes.

Spinal anesthetic: Generally used for surgical anesthesia. Like an epidural, this regional block innervates the uterus. *Upside*: Instead of requiring a catheter, it is a one-shot-and-done option. It's a good choice for a mom delivering by Caesarean section (C-section). It is a very safe form of anesthesia but used in a different context than an epidural. *Downside*: It's not meant for long-term anesthesia and usually only lasts one to two hours.

Caudal, saddle, and pudendal blocks: These numbing shots affect the outlet of the birth canal. *Upside*: Useful when you're at the "ring of fire" stage and the pain is just too intense to manage or in an emergency delivery situation. *Downside*: Not long-lasting, though at the point they'd be given, you wouldn't need them to be.

General anesthetic: This type is less common today but may be used for an emergency C-section or other emergency birth situations when there is not enough time to place an epidural or administer spinal anesthesia. *Upside*: Heck, if your doctor and anesthesiologist conclude you need a general anesthetic and it's the safest course of action, then hooray that it exists. *Downside*: You will be asleep for the delivery, and the meds cross the placenta and can have a sedative effect on the baby after birth.

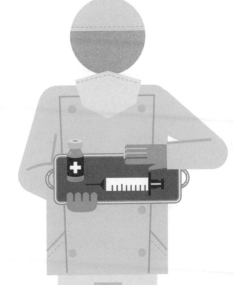

Tips from the Trenches: Energy Conservation and the Laboring Mom

There are many things your friends who've given birth may not think to warn you about before the big day. Just remember, you too will pretty much forget all the nitty-gritty details after a year or so. Meantime, take heed of some basic advice for getting yourself through labor:

[1] Don't forget to eat! You wouldn't go on a day-long mountain climb without calorie intake, so labor should be no different. You will need energy for all the hard work that lies ahead.

[2] Don't overdo the eating, however. The uterus is a giant muscle that is contracting regularly and taking all the oxygen and nutrients to do its job, so if you eat a lot or eat heavy food, it will not be properly digested and can make you nauseated. Another reason to avoid a double cheeseburger: If the need arises for a C-section, you do not want to be at risk for vomiting and aspiration, which can be a life-threatening complication for you (not the baby).

[3] Eat and drink what feels good: granola bars, soup, pasta, crackers, water, sports drinks. If you know your practitioner forbids food intake once you are admitted, eat something on the car ride or in the elevator to labor and delivery.

[4] Stick to clear fluids and things like ice chips and lollipops once labor has begun.

[5] Stay hydrated. Birthing requires lots of fluids.

[6] Take it easy when you are pushing during Stage 2:

■ Push through the contraction as your body dictates.
■ Relax your face and unclench your teeth. The muscles in your face aren't going to get the baby out, so push from below. (This will also minimize broken blood vessels in your eyes and face.)
■ Don't hold your breath. Keep oxygen flowing to the baby. He's going through this labor, too.

Getting a Little or a Lot of Help with Delivery

Whether you are delivering at home, a birthing center, or a hospital, the goal is to have a healthy baby and a healthy mom. Under ideal circumstances, that happens without any medical interventions.

But with some deliveries, quick action may be required to ensure a healthy outcome. Some scenarios your practitioner will already know about prior to labor, including breach or transverse fetal position, overly large baby, dwindling amniotic fluid, placenta previa, or postdate pregnancy; others arise only during labor, such as passed meconium, fetal distress, a dropped heart rate, shoulder dystocia, arrested progress, or maternal exhaustion.

Rest assured that your practitioner knows what to do in each of these scenarios. Here are some of the methods he or she may use to make sure labor progresses:

Stripping the membrane: This process separates the amniotic sac from the cervix, releasing prostaglandins that soften the cervix and cause contractions.

Ripening the cervix: The cervix is like a peach. When unripe it is hard and firm, and when it ripens it gets soft and mushy and pliable to dilation. Medicines containing prostaglandins ripen the cervix, which then leads to labor.

Amniotomy: A long plastic hook called an amniohook is inserted, breaking the amniotic sac. Now baby's head can put direct pressure on the cervix to soften and thin it, speeding dilation.

Induction: If you are post due or need to get labor going before your body begins on its own; or if labor is stalling (and baby may be experiencing distress or diminished oxygen supply), you can be placed on an IV Pitocin drip, a synthetic version of a natural hormone called oxytocin, to induce labor contractions.

Episiotomy: This surgical procedure allows additional room for the baby's head to crown and move faster out of the birth canal, particularly if there are concerns about baby's oxygen supply. After a local anesthetic is given to numb the perineal area, scissors are used to make a neat cut at varying levels through tissue from the vaginal opening toward the anus. This incision controls the potential for tearing.

✚ DOC TALK: *I tell patients that about 90 percent of women will have stitches from the baby coming through the birth canal, whether from an episiotomy or from a tear. Although there are recommendations against routine episiotomy, in certain situations it may be safer for Mom and/or baby. It is impossible to predict who might need this procedure until the moment of delivery of the baby's head. I try to steer patients away from absolute refusals. Absolutes are dangerous in such a dynamic environment, where so many variables can change in moments.*

Forceps or vacuum extraction: These tools help move the baby out of the birth canal. When progress has stalled despite Mom's efforts, and depending on the baby's position and the degree of descent in the birth canal, it may be safer for the doctor to assist pushing with gentle pulling, using either forceps or vacuum. Forceps are like big spoons that are placed around the baby's head. The doctor can pull on the handle of the spoons to assist delivery. Vacuum extraction works the same way, but with a small suction cup placed on top of the baby's head, with a handle that allows the doctor to assist. An episiotomy is usually performed to make room for the forceps or vacuum. These devices may be used when the baby is in distress and an urgent delivery is necessary. These tools sound scary (not to mention the mental pictures dancing around in your head), but when used properly they can be life-saving interventions and may also help you avoid a Caesarian section.

Caesarian section: Also called a C-section, this major surgical procedure is performed in the operating room. After you receive an epidural, spinal, or general anesthesia (if there is not time to administer an epidural), the surgeon will make an incision usually transversely along the bikini line, and then another incision in the uterus to extract the baby and the placenta. You will have a dull sensation of tugging and pulling, but no pain. Your partner can typically be present, stationed by your head and wearing sterile surgical scrubs. A screen will drape your and your partner's view of the operation, but you will be alert for the entire procedure if you've had an epidural or spinal. Postoperatively, you'll need more time to recover in the hospital than women who deliver vaginally.

DOC TALK: One thing we monitor to assess how a baby is tolerating labor is the fetal heart rate. This is analogous to your going to the doctor and the only thing she could check to see if you were okay was your pulse—that is, not a very good indicator! Today, with C-sections being straightforward and relatively safe, if the heart rate is suspicious, I recommend that you do not take a chance with the health of your baby.

Capturing the Moment

Don't forget to take a picture of the big finale. Whether you have an elaborate digital camera, an old film-loading one, or a disposable model, you will definitely want to have it handy. A few hints:

[1] Make sure you haven't packed your camera at the bottom of your suitcase.

[2] Pick up a disposable camera in case yours jams, loses its charge, falls in the toilet, etc.

[3] You may even want to discuss with your partner ahead of time just what you want to be captured for posterity, and what not:

■ Do you want your partner present, holding your hand for baby's arrival, or poised to snap a picture? (Maybe a nurse could grab the camera so your partner can be close to you and not fiddling with equipment.)
■ Do you want the event recorded on video?
■ Will this moment be something you want to relive over and over or something you would simply prefer to recall orally? It may be too graphic for some more modest moms, and you should consider whether you want your child popping the footage into the DVD player by accident later. Good ol' scientific reality—or scary horror show of Mom's privates? Let your lifestyle and personality dictate that choice.

[4] Finally, don't forget to enlist one of the nurses to take a group shot of the happy family once everything has settled down. Try not to end up with a snapshot of you, the baby, and the doula. Make sure Dad makes it into the picture!

⚠️ **EXPERT TIP:** *If you forget the camera, don't sweat it. You'll have a lifetime of chances to photograph your cute little baby growing up and doing a thousand amazing things.*

⚠️ **JUST FOR DADS:** *Labor, delivery, and birth are an incredible physical and emotional journey for both you and Mom. We often see dads moved to tears at the first sight of their son or daughter, then sometimes confused as moms need time to regroup after such a long ordeal. Be prepared for conflicting emotions. Labor is painful, so don't be put off if Mom needs some time to herself to regroup before sharing in the joy.*

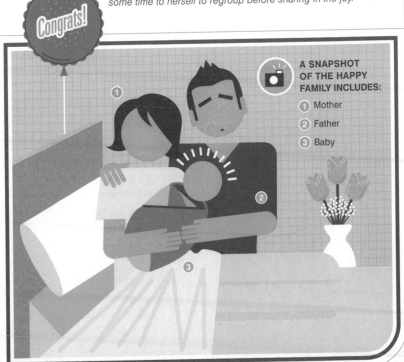

Congrats!

A SNAPSHOT OF THE HAPPY FAMILY INCLUDES:

1. Mother
2. Father
3. Baby

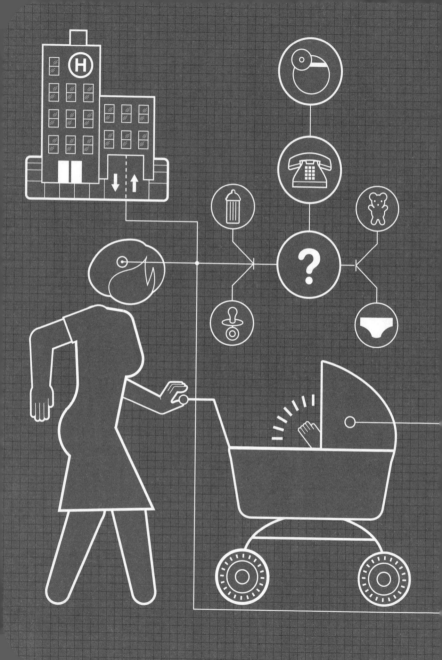

Chapter 8

Baby on Board

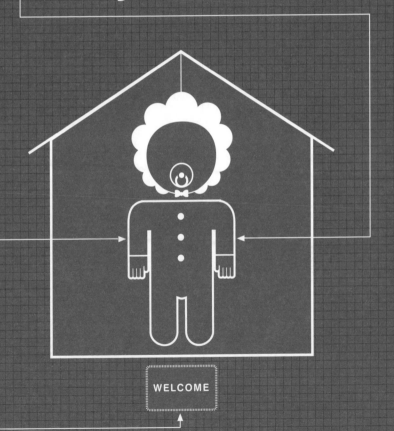

WELCOME

Once your son or daughter arrives you may be so exhausted and so happy that you don't even notice the whirl of activities surrounding you and your baby. If possible, take a moment to savor this time: Here's your child! He's finally here! This is a heady, exciting moment. Don't be surprised, however, to see the medical personnel bustling about in a no-nonsense way to make sure baby is tolerating his arrival into the world.

Every hospital or birthing center has its own way of doing things, but this chapter details some standard measures you can expect. (Of course, if you are birthing at home, these procedures will differ, with much of the medical screening taking place some days after the birth, at the pediatrician's office.)

Welcome to the World, Baby!

A few procedures are pro forma after delivery and happen rapidly. Rest assured, the nurses will keep in close contact with you even as they put baby through the paces. While you are being tended to and made more comfortable after your exertions, the following will take place.

Suction: The baby's nose and mouth will be suctioned with a bulb syringe after her head emerges from the vaginal canal. Your nurse may request that you stop pushing for a moment so she can perform the suctioning. (After your baby is completely delivered and the umbilical cord is clamped and cut, she will receive a second suction.)

Tummy time: Your baby will be placed tummy to tummy with you immediately after birth, so the fluids can continue to drain from your baby and you have some instant skin-to-skin contact with your little one.

Cut umbilical cord: Usually Dad or your significant other will cut the cord after it has been clamped on either side of the place where the cut will occur. If you are birthing naturally, you may want to wait a few moments before cutting the cord to allow additional blood flow and give baby an extra boost after delivery. (Note, however, that there are some situations—such as passed meconium or if the baby is unresponsive—when it is beneficial to clamp and cut quickly and hand the baby right over to the waiting pediatricians.) The small stump remaining will be trimmed and capped with a plastic clamp, then sterilized with Triple Dye, Betadine, or another antibacterial agent. For the next week or ten days (until the stump falls off), you will be cleaning the stump with each diaper change. Your nurse or midwife will show you how.

EXPERT TIP: During a C-section, Dad will not be able to cut the cord since the operating field is sterile and you do not want to introduce contamination while Mom's belly is exposed. In these cases, Dad will usually be able to trim the cord at the baby warmer so that he still gets the experience.

Apgar score: Named for anesthesiologist Virginia Apgar, this standardized measure for assessing your newborn's well-being is conducted at one minute after birth and then again at five minutes after birth. Your doctor will observe your baby's heart rate, breathing, muscle tone, reflex response, and color, rating each measure with a number between zero (lowest) and two (highest).

DOC TALK: Many parents worry when their child does not get a perfect Apgar score, but infants (even your OB's children!) rarely score a perfect ten. One point may be taken off for color (most blood flow is going to her vital organs first, so baby's hands and feet will usually stay blue even up to 24 hours, until her whole system is up and running) or for respiration (many babies will take time to cry at first because, like Mom, they have also had quite a journey and may be tuckered out).

Breast-feeding: If you have decided to breast-feed, you will be given your newborn for immediate postpartum feeding. Even if she feeds only briefly, she will "imprint" on you at this time, facilitating later breast-feeding. The added benefit: It will also help your uterus contract and deliver the placenta. Your doula or nurse will help you get into the position that allows your baby to nurse.

Physical exam: Your baby will get a head-to-toe exam. He will be weighed and, eventually, measured (after he gets the chance to stretch out and relax from his curled-up fetal position). Note: If your baby weighs less than 5½ pounds (2.5 kg), he will be considered "low birth weight" and will receive special attention immediately and thereafter in the nursery. Also, big babies (more than 9 pounds [4 kg]) will get extra care in respect to their weight and calorie intake. These infants tend to use up their sugar stores quickly and may need to feed immediately or be supplemented with a bottle.

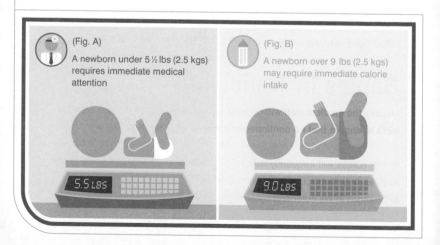

(Fig. A) A newborn under 5 ½ lbs (2.5 kgs) requires immediate medical attention

(Fig. B) A newborn over 9 lbs (2.5 kgs) may require immediate calorie intake

5.5 LBS

9.0 LBS

Ophthalmic antibiotics: The nurse will apply an ophthalmic antibiotic ointment to your baby's eyes as a prophylactic to prevent the transmission of gonorrhea to the baby. (Gonorrhea is a devastating infection that can cause blindness, so antibiotics are administered as a universal procedure.)

Footprints and bracelets: Baby's footprints will be taken, and for security purposes matching identification bracelets will be placed on your baby and you and your partner. (These are good mementos of your stay; years and even months later you will be astonished at how tiny your baby's anklet was!)

Vitamin K shot: Babies are born without vitamin K, a nutrient that assists in blood clotting, so a vitamin K shot gives them a head start until their bodies can house sufficient quantities to prevent (rare) haemorrhagic disease of the newborn (HDN).

Blood draw: Some babies may need a blood test to make sure they are not hypoglycemic. Blood is typically drawn from the heel. Also, babies born to moms with certain blood types will also be tested to ensure that baby's blood does not have antigens that will act against his own red blood cells.

Babies in Transition

Usually the medical staff will observe your baby for up to four hours after birth to ensure that he continues to tolerate life outside the womb.

- The nurses will frequently assess your baby's respiratory rate, temperature, and cardiovascular function.
- Changes in his color and breathing will be monitored.

■ If your baby was delivered by C-section, he might have respiratory problems: Unlike babies born vaginally, the amniotic fluid will not have been squeezed out of his lungs during the trip through the birth canal. The staff will check to see that any residual amniotic fluid dries up in his first few days of life.

■ Your baby will be bathed and swaddled.

■ Once you and your partner give consent, a hepatitis B vaccine will be administered (perhaps not immediately, but at some point before you and baby are discharged).

Baby's First Tests

She's just a few hours old, and already she's taking exams! Depending on how quickly you and your newborn will be discharged from your caregiver (ranging from one to two days for vaginal delivery to five days for C-sections), the following tests will be conducted during your stay.

[1] Your newborn will have his blood drawn to screen for various disorders, including hypothyroidism; hemoglobinopathies; endocrine, amino acid, urea cycle, fatty acid oxidation and organic acid disorders; and biotinidase deficiency. The blood will be sent to the lab and results will be sent to the parents, the hospital, and the newborn's pediatrician. (Make sure the hospital has your pediatrician's name and address.) This screening has also been referred to as a PKU test since it screens for that amino acid disorder, but it is now a much broader safeguard.

[2] Your newborn will have her hearing screened. Set off in a quiet area, she will wear tiny headphones, and the administrator will look for her responses to sound levels.

[3] If your baby is jaundiced or yellowish, it may be that she has a condition called hyperbilirubinemia, which occurs when the baby's liver has difficulty eliminating bilirubin (a breakdown product of used red blood cells that, until now, has been dealt with by the placenta). A screening for bilirubin ensures that baby avoids any neurologic effects. If her levels are high, she may require simple phototherapy: She will be exposed to lights that will help decrease the jaundice.

Postdelivery FAQs

Now that you and baby have settled in for some rest after your extremely exhausting day, you begin to set the stage for the routines that will continue once both go home. Here's what to expect postdelivery if you are recovering in a hospital setting.

[1] You will have the choice of "rooming in" with baby (see page 209) or having her cared for by nursing staff, at least some of the time, in the newborn nursery.

[2] Nurses will take baby's vital signs and periodically assess his well-being, checking weight and ensuring that he has no postpartum problems. (Remember that babies lose weight in the first few days before adding it back on; ideally, his weight should not dip below a 10 percent weight loss from birth weight.)

[3] If you have chosen to breast-feed, you will now be getting into the nursing rhythm of feeding your baby every two to three hours. (See page 211 for more details.) If you are remaining in the hospital for several days, take advantage of breast-feeding classes that typically meet on the maternity ward.

[4] Many hospitals offer a class that covers the basics of newborn care (how to bathe baby, diapering, cord care, circumcision care, etc.). Ask your nurse if such a class exists and when and where it takes place. Attending will help you gear up for your first few days at home—when you realize you're truly a parent!

[5] If you and your partner choose to circumcise, you may have your baby's pediatrician or your obstetrician perform the procedure while you and your son are still in the hospital. (Some parents may want to wait until later, to comply with religious tradition.) The doctor can use a local anesthetic block at the base of the penis, a sugar nipple that essentially blisses out the baby with glucose, or some numbing cream at the incision site. Follow-up care of the incision is easy: Keep it covered with petroleum jelly or A&D ointment. It will take about a week to heal.

[6] Many birthing facilities provide newborn photo services that allow you to share photos of your little one just days after she was born.

[7] There's no law that says your baby must leave the hospital with a name, but for practical reasons it can be helpful to have a completed birth certificate put into process by hospital staff (along with other official documents), instead of having to chase down the paperwork afterward.

Rooming In

When your baby stays with you in the hospital room, you are doing what's known as "rooming in." Your infant must be cleared medically (most are), but mothers are encouraged to keep their babies in the room as much as possible, even sleeping in the room overnight.

■ If you need some time to yourself to get some solid rest, the baby can always return to the nursery.

■ Overnight bonding is especially useful if you are breast-feeding. Prolactin is a hormone that stimulates milk production and it peaks at night, so if you capitalize on your increased prolactin and baby's natural evening alertness, chances are you will get your breast-feeding off to a better start.

■ If you are worried you will sleep through your baby's cries for food, don't be. Mothers are tuned into their baby's cries and movement—as you'll soon find out!

■ Remember to sleep when the baby sleeps so you can harness your energy appropriately. Save entertaining visitors, friends, and family for later.

■ If you are breast-feeding and worried that if your baby spends time in the nursery he will get a bottle, don't be. Just clarify your wishes with the nurses.

■ The hospital stay is about rest and recovery, so don't feel guilty about taking lots of naps. You will need all the energy you can get to be ready to take care of your newborn at home.

Remember these hints when you return home as well. Many moms are tempted to use the time when baby is sleeping to tidy up, do errands, and write thank-you notes for baby gifts. *Don't*. After you put the baby down, put yourself down as well. If you wake up before the baby does, then use any of that leftover time to do those tasks on your list. You need to get as much sleep as possible to function at your best!

⚠ **EXPERT TIP:** *Rooming in is also a great time to do some "kangarooing," a technique that promotes parent-baby bonding. Your baby has spent the last nine months in utero, so he won't want to be separated from you (that will come in about 13 more years). Instead of wrapping him up and plunking him in a plastic crib across the room, try taking off everything except his diaper and cuddle him next to your bare skin. Once you are skin to skin, put a blanket over the baby. Hearing Mom's heartbeat and voice and smelling her skin will keep baby happy. When he's hungry he will root his way over to your breast. Plus, your body temperature will help regulate the baby's temperature. Dads are encouraged to do this, too, for bonding and to enhance baby's sense of security.*

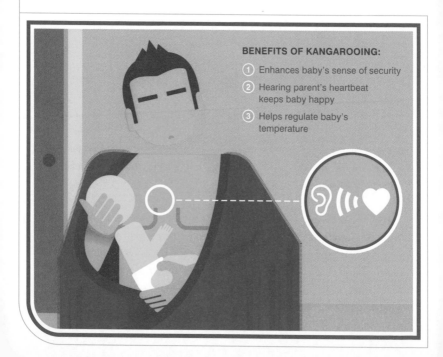

BENEFITS OF KANGAROOING:

1. Enhances baby's sense of security
2. Hearing parent's heartbeat keeps baby happy
3. Helps regulate baby's temperature

Time to Feed the Baby

If you opt to breast-feed, which is recommended by pediatricians, the baby will begin to nurse immediately. From a medical standpoint, immediate breast-feeding is beneficial to both Mom and child. The suckling stimulates the release of oxytocin from the brain, which helps contract the uterus and minimize bleeding. Some facts to be aware of:

■ Initially, you will produce colostrum. This thick, yellowish liquid is dense in calories, nutrients, and protective maternal antibodies.

■ Some babies may not immediately exhibit strong interest in feeding. Many babies will continue to cough and sneeze and have a runny nose for the first day or two as they clear the remnants of amniotic fluid from their lungs. When ready, they will demonstrate the rooting reflex by turning their head to the side and making gnawing motions with their mouth. Get ready!

■ After a few days of nursing, your milk will "come in," and you may feel what's called a "let-down response" signaling that your body's milk supply is ready.

■ Babies should be fed on demand, usually every two or three hours.

■ In the beginning, your little one will spend up to a half-hour on each breast.

■ Many breast-feeding women worry that they will not have adequate supply, but usually it is simply a matter of working out the mom and child's supply-and-demand system.

■ If your baby loses more than 10 percent of his birth weight, you may choose to supplement with formula. Once baby's weight is stable, resume strictly breast-feeding.

■ Bottle-fed babies should be fed on demand as well, but they will not need to be fed as often since formula takes longer to digest than breast milk. One of the best things about bottle feeding is that Mom can get a break from the round-the-clock feedings and minimize her sleep deprivation by having Dad or another caregiver get up to feed the baby.

EXPERT TIP: *Most moms will require the guidance of nurses or lactation specialists to help with breast-feeding issues such as latching on, positioning, engorgement, and nipple soreness. Many hospitals and birthing centers will offer classes before you leave and some type of call line to answer breast-feeding questions once you get home. (Prenatal breast-feeding classes are also highly recommended.)*

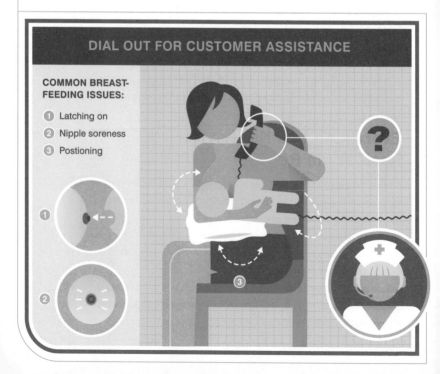

Home, Baby!

Preparing to leave the hospital or birthing center can be a truly exciting time—perhaps tinged with some anxiety. On one hand, you can't wait to get your baby home and to be home yourself. But on the other hand, it sure has been nice to have a full-time staff of baby and new-mom experts around to instruct and care for you.

Rest assured, millions of moms have shared your anxieties and even gone on to do this amazing adventure again and again. Meantime, your caregivers will be sure to help you put your best foot forward:

■ In many facilities, your doctor will write orders for your discharge, and a nurse will go over your and your baby's postpartum care instructions, including recuperation guidelines for those recovering from C-sections and episiotomies.

■ Most facilities will escort you and your child out to your car, which of course you've already equipped with a newborn car seat.

Everything You Need to Know About Postpartum Recovery

Restricted activities: After a vaginal delivery the cervix takes time to close, so to prevent infection of the uterus most doctors will restrict your activities (no intercourse, tub baths, or swimming) until the postpartum checkup, usually four to six weeks after delivery.

Stitches: Most women will have some stitches in the perineal area, which will usually dissolve in about a week or two. You can expect to see small amounts of suture material when you use toilet tissue. Not to worry. This is supposed to happen as the sutures break down and fall out.

Pain: Anticipate having pain and discomfort for at least two weeks. Passing a baby through the birth canal irritates the nerves along the spine and hips and stretches and tears many of the pelvic support muscles. These will need time to heal. Many moms will notice that they have shoulder and leg pains and even numbness in the lower extremities from the pressure the baby's head put on the related nerves. This discomfort is normal and will resolve in the days and weeks following delivery.

Swelling: The body holds on to an incredible amount of water during pregnancy. After the baby comes, your body begins to mobilize this fluid, and it will take about two weeks to pee out the majority. During this time you can expect significant swelling, especially in your ankles and feet. The peak of the swelling occurs once you're home. (Note: If one leg is significantly more swollen than the other, you may be at risk of developing a blood clot and you should contact your doctor immediately; small differences are nothing to worry about.)

Bleeding: After delivery, postpartum bleeding, known as locchia, will be heavy. It will slowly taper off, but there is no right schedule for when it will stop entirely. Some women will stop bleeding in a few days and then see irregular bleeding over the next couple weeks. Others have constant, low levels of bleeding. If the bleeding is persistently heavy or if you are passing clots bigger than an apple, call your doctor to make sure everything is okay.

Menstrual changes: When you breast-feed, you suppress estrogen production, which means most breast-feeding moms will not experience a menstrual period. You may have light, irregular bleeding but no regular menses. That is normal. But be warned: You can still get pregnant. So make sure you address birth control with your doctor, unless you intend to become pregnant while still changing your infant's diapers.

Bladder control: After you deliver your baby, your pelvic muscles and, hence, your bladder will sit a bit lower, which may give you an uncomfortable feeling of pressure. Any increase in pressure, such as from coughing, laughing, and sneezing, can cause an unwanted release of urine. This sitation should improve as the bladder and pelvic muscles regain their tone. Kegel exercises will speed the process of getting your muscles back into shape (see page 68).

Abdominal stretching: Saggy tummies are another reason for postpartum woe. Abdominal muscles have been stretched during months and months of pregnancy, so they will not tighten in four to six weeks. By the postpartum checkup, these muscles may be in much better shape, but it typically takes several months for moms to achieve prepregnancy fitness levels.

C-section recovery: Postoperative instructions are much the same as for vaginal births. You may have some additional restrictions on lifting heavy objects to avoid stressing the incision and to allow proper healing. In general, it's wise to avoid lifting anything over 30–40 pounds (13.5–18 kg). Stairs are okay if taken slowly. Many moms need to be able to pick up their older children, so you have to do what you have to do without overdoing it. Anticipate some back and forth of good days and bad days in the first two weeks as your body begins to heal.

You're Somebody's Mom

Once you and your baby are at home, your new life begins. Things will never be the same. That means in a very ordinary don't-forget-to-buy-diapers, go-to-bed-by-10 P.M., swap-burping-techniques way and also in the big, dramatic chord-playing cosmic way. You now have a stake in the world like never before. World politics, the environment, religion, family life, cultural traditions . . . the list goes on. There is something profound and humbling about being the shepherd of a new person and feeling that responsibility down to your marrow as you rock him to sleep while he listens to your heartbeat. This tiny miracle in your arms is effortlessly and completely dependent on you, and you're shaping the world and his expectations of it. At least initially.

Here's another mind-bending truth. For many new moms, time will pass like molasses. Around 11 A.M., it will feel like time to start making supper. (Beginning your day at 4:30 A.M. will do that.) You'll run through your bag of tricks to amuse your baby. Then you will look again at the time and find it discouraging that only seven minutes have passed.

How will you ever survive the pacing of this new time flow? Check in again when your child is five years old, and the time will seem to have fast-forwarded. Consider the feeling when your kindergartner loses her first tooth. That's the tooth you remember crowing over with triumph when it boldly crept up beyond the gum line of your baby, leading the charge for the other 19 to follow.

Cherish this remarkable period when babies are dimpled and sweet as sugar. For sure, there will be other pleasures along the way, as they grow into interesting adults. But this time of being new parents, when everything is fresh, exhausting, and astonishing, is precious. Embrace its silly, confusing newness and the fact that your heartburn has vanished—at least until you decide to make some brothers and sisters and start this whole process all over again.

And know this: All those grannies who come up to you in the park and say, "Enjoy this time. It passes in a blink of the eye"—they're right.

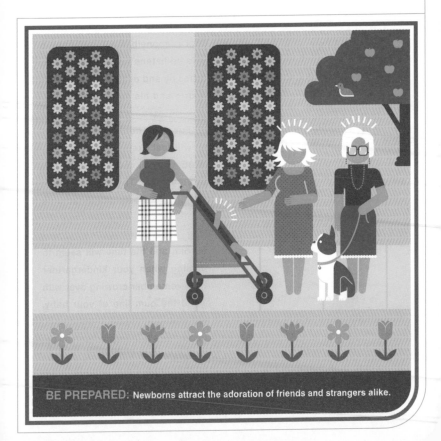

BE PREPARED: Newborns attract the adoration of friends and strangers alike.

Index

About the Authors

SARAH JORDAN is a National Magazine Award–nominated author who has written for magazines and newspapers including *Parents*, *Parenting*, *Philadelphia Magazine*, and *The Philadelphia Inquirer*. She is also the coauthor of *The Worst-Case Scenario Survival Handbook: Parenting* and *The Worst-Case Scenario Survival Handbook: Weddings*. She lives in Philadelphia with her husband and two children.

DAVID UFBERG, M.D., is a practicing obstetrician and gynecologist at Pennsylvania Hospital in Philadelphia. An assistant clinical professor with the University of Pennsylvania Health System, he has written several research publications and received many teaching awards. He is a devoted husband and father of three and has delivered thousands of babies.

About the Illustrators

PAUL KEPPLE and SCOTTY REIFSNYDER are better known as the Philadelphia-based studio HEADCASE DESIGN. Their work has been featured in many design and illustration publications, such as *AIGA 365* and *50 Books/50 Covers, American Illustration*, *Communication Arts*, and *Print*. Paul worked at Running Press Book Publishers for several years before opening Headcase in 1998. Paul graduated from the Tyler School of Art, where he now teaches. Scotty is a graduate of Kutztown University and received his M.F.A. from Tyler School of Art, where he had Paul as an instructor. Scotty's mother claims he came close to having a brilliant career as a TV baby, but his lack of comic timing kept him on the casting couch. Paul's mother also thought he should have been a TV baby, but unfortunately no one else agreed.